WALL PILATES FOR SENIORS TO LOSE WEIGHT

Empowering Fitness & Sustainable Weight Management Through Gentle Movement

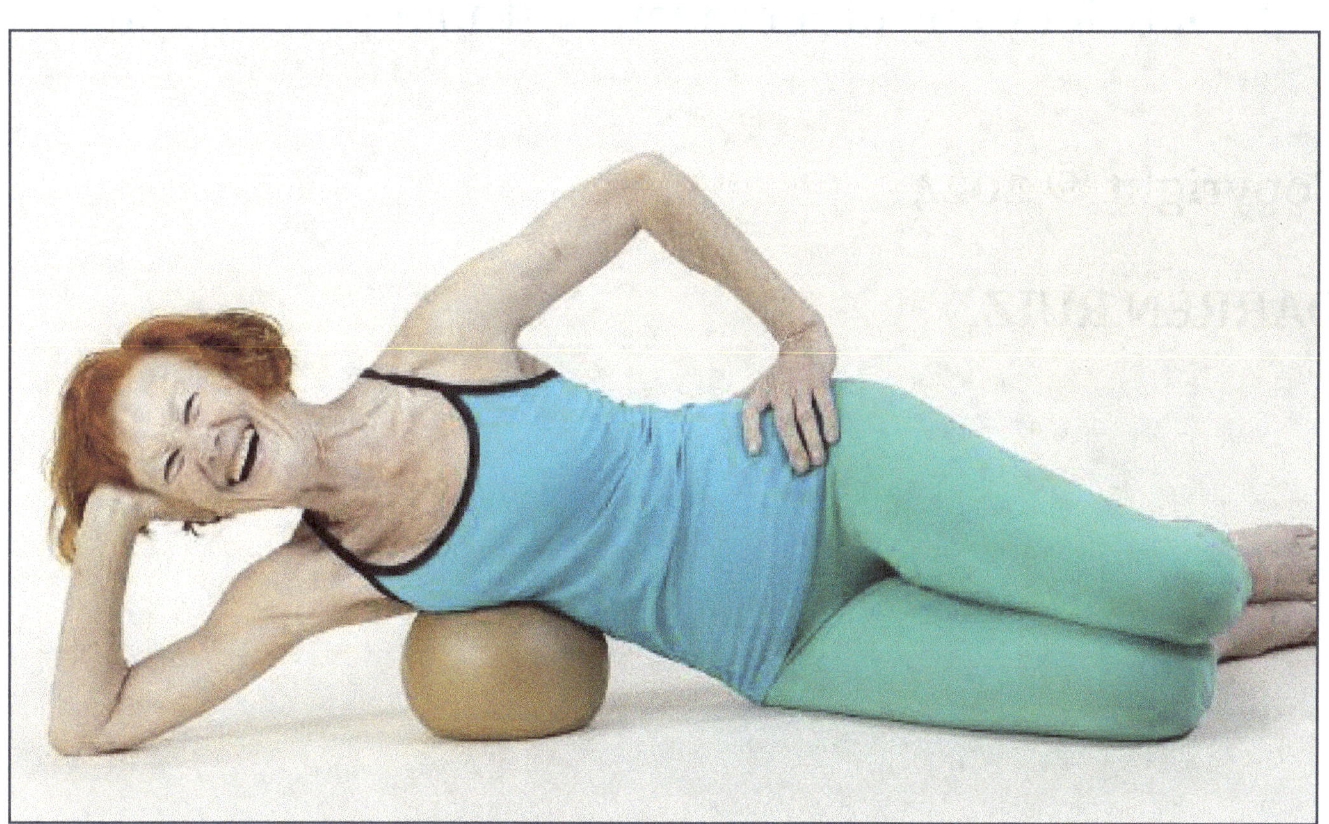

DARREN RUIZ

<u>Disclaimer</u>

The information provided in this book is for general informational and educational purposes only and is not a substitute for professional medical advice, diagnosis, or treatment. Always consult with a qualified healthcare professional before starting any new exercise program, especially if you have any pre-existing health conditions or concerns. The exercises and recommendations in this book are intended for seniors with a basic level of fitness and mobility. If you experience any pain or discomfort while performing these exercises, stop immediately and seek medical attention. The author and publisher of this book disclaim any liability or loss in connection with the exercises and advice herein.

Contents

WALL PILATES FOR SENIORS TO LOSE WEIGHT

INTRODUCTION

Overview of Wall Pilates

Wall Pilates is a gentle, yet effective form of exercise tailored specifically for seniors, offering a perfect blend of strength, flexibility, and balance. This low-impact workout utilizes a wall as a supportive tool, making it accessible and safe for individuals of all fitness levels.

The versatility of Wall Pilates is among its most alluring features. Exercises can be modified to suit individual needs, ensuring that everyone, regardless of their physical condition, can participate and benefit. This inclusivity fosters a sense of community and belonging, which is crucial for seniors who often face isolation.

The simplicity of Wall Pilates is its charm. The wall provides a stable surface, reducing the risk of falls and injuries. This stability allows seniors to focus on their movements, enhancing their body awareness and improving posture. As they progress, they experience increased strength, particularly in the core muscles, which are essential for maintaining balance and preventing falls.

Wall Pilates also offers a unique opportunity for seniors to reconnect with their bodies. The slow, controlled movements encourage mindfulness, helping them tune into their physical sensations and breathe more effectively. This mind-body connection is not only beneficial for physical health but also for mental well-being, reducing stress and promoting relaxation.

Moreover, Wall Pilates can be a fun and social activity. Group classes provide a chance to meet new people, share experiences, and support each other's fitness journeys. The sense of achievement and camaraderie that comes from practicing Wall Pilates together can be incredibly motivating and rewarding.

In conclusion, Wall Pilates is an excellent choice for seniors looking to improve their fitness in a safe, supportive, and enjoyable way. Its adaptability, focus on balance and strength, and the opportunity for social interaction make it a workout that seniors will not only benefit from but also fall in love with and look forward to.

Benefits of Wall Pilates for Seniors

Wall Pilates offers a multitude of benefits for seniors, particularly in the realm of weight loss and overall well-being. Here's a list of core benefits:

1. **Low-Impact Exercise:** Wall Pilates is gentle on the joints, making it an ideal form of exercise for seniors who may have arthritis or other joint issues.

2. **Weight Loss:** By engaging multiple muscle groups, Wall Pilates can help burn calories and promote weight loss, which is crucial for maintaining a healthy weight and reducing the risk of obesity-related health issues.

3. **Improved Balance and Stability:** The exercises focus on core strength, which is essential for balance and stability, reducing the risk of falls and injuries.

4. **Enhanced Flexibility:** Wall Pilates helps increase flexibility, which can improve range of motion and reduce stiffness and pain in the muscles and joints.

5. **Better Posture:** Regular practice of Wall Pilates can lead to improved posture, which can alleviate back pain and other posture-related issues.

6. **Increased Muscle Strength:** The exercises target various muscle groups, leading to increased overall strength, which is vital for daily activities and independence.

7. **Stress Reduction:** The mindful nature of Wall Pilates, combined with controlled breathing, can help reduce stress and promote relaxation.

8. **Improved Cardiovascular Health:** While primarily a strength-based exercise, Wall Pilates can also have cardiovascular benefits, improving heart health and circulation.

9. **Enhanced Mind-Body Connection:** Practicing Wall Pilates encourages mindfulness and body awareness, leading to a better understanding of one's body and its needs.

10. **Social Interaction:** Joining a Wall Pilates class can provide social interaction and a sense of community, which is important for mental health and well-being.

By incorporating Wall Pilates into their routine, seniors can enjoy these benefits, leading to a healthier, more active lifestyle and effective weight management.

Why Wall Pilates

For seniors seeking an effective and sustainable approach to weight loss, Wall Pilates presents a compelling solution. This form of exercise stands out for its unique combination of accessibility, safety, and efficacy, making it particularly well-suited for older adults.

One of the key reasons to adopt Wall Pilates is its low-impact nature. Unlike high-intensity workouts that can be harsh on aging joints, Wall Pilates provides a gentle yet effective way to burn calories and shed excess weight. The exercises are designed to be performed with the support of a wall, which not only aids in balance but also ensures proper alignment and reduces the risk of injury. This makes it an ideal choice for seniors who may have concerns about falls or joint pain.

Moreover, Wall Pilates focuses on building core strength, which is crucial for overall stability and balance. A strong core not only supports a healthy posture but also enhances the body's ability to perform everyday activities more efficiently, leading to increased calorie burn even outside of exercise sessions. The emphasis on controlled, mindful movements also means that practitioners are more likely to engage muscles effectively, maximizing the workout's benefits for weight loss.

In addition to its physical advantages, Wall Pilates offers mental benefits that can support weight loss goals. The practice encourages mindfulness and stress reduction, which are important factors in managing emotional eating and maintaining a healthy relationship with food. By promoting a sense of calm and focus, Wall Pilates can help seniors navigate the psychological aspects of weight loss with greater ease.

In summary, Wall Pilates provides a holistic approach to weight loss for seniors, addressing both physical and mental well-being. Its low-impact, core-focused exercises offer a safe and efficient way to achieve and maintain a healthy weight, making it an excellent choice for older adults looking to enhance their fitness and overall quality of life.

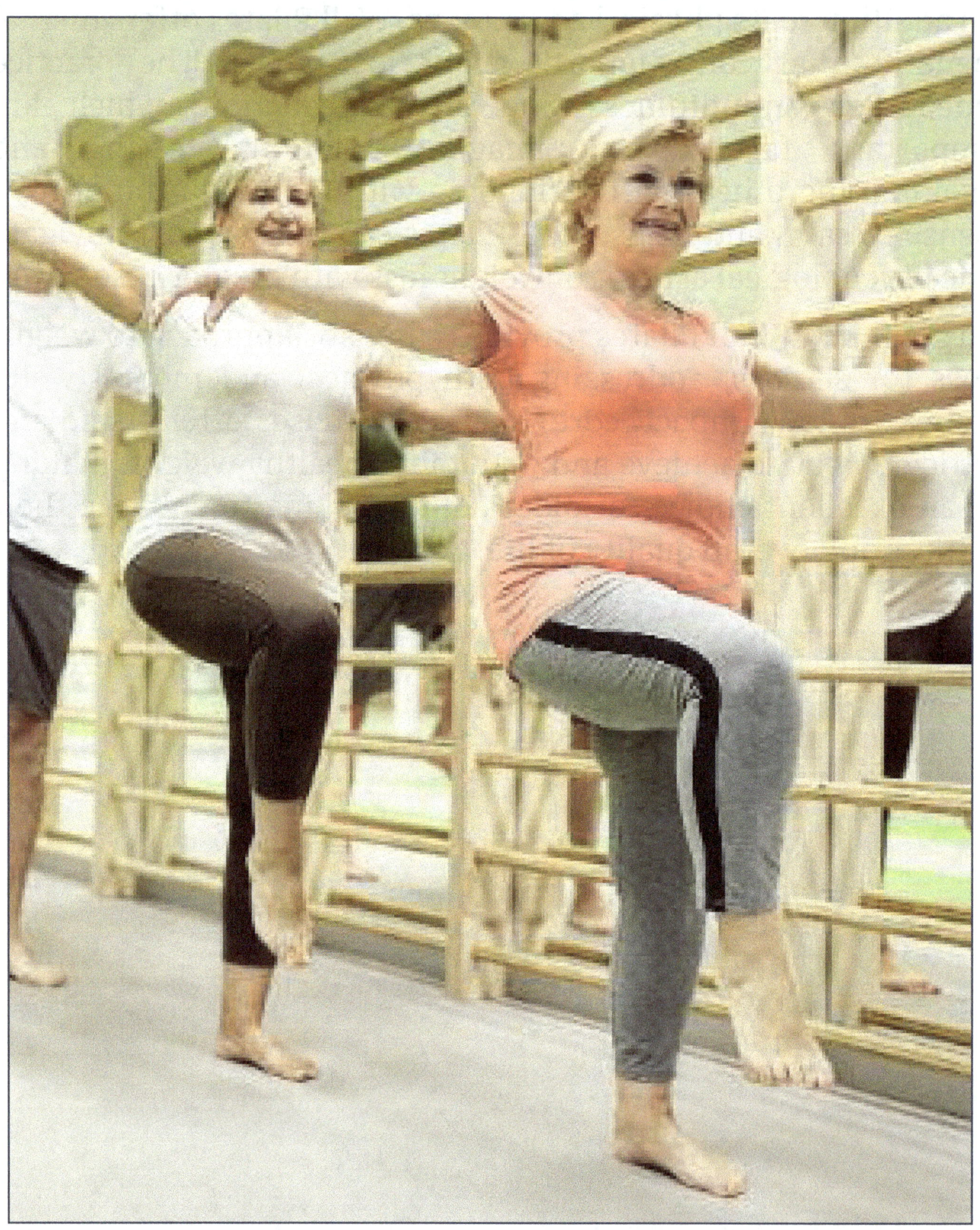

WALL PILATES FOR SENIORS TO LOSE WEIGHT

SETTING UP FOR SUCCESS

Creating a Safe and Comfortable Practice Area at Home

Creating a safe and comfortable practice area at home is crucial for seniors engaging in Wall Pilates. Here are some guidelines to ensure a conducive environment for your workouts:

1. **Choose the Right Floor Surface:** opt for a non-slip surface to prevent falls during your exercises. A yoga mat or a Pilates mat can provide cushioning and grip, making it safer and more comfortable for your practice. If you have carpeted floors, ensure the carpet is firmly attached and not too thick, as this can affect your balance.
2. **Select a Suitable Wall:** The wall you choose should be sturdy and free of obstructions like paintings or shelves. Ensure its smooth and clean to prevent any injuries. If you're using a painted wall, make sure the paint is not slippery.
3. **Ensure Adequate Space:** You should have enough room to move freely without bumping into furniture. A clear space of at least 6 feet by 3 feet is recommended. This will allow you to perform a range of movements without restriction.
4. **Lighting and Ventilation:** Good lighting is essential for visibility and safety. Natural light is ideal, but if that's not possible, ensure your practice area is well-lit with artificial lights. Proper ventilation is also important to keep the air fresh and prevent overheating.

5. **Wear Appropriate Clothing:** Choose comfortable, breathable clothing that allows for a full range of motion. Avoid loose clothing that could get caught or restrict your movements. Supportive footwear or non-slip socks can provide additional stability, especially if you have balance concerns.

6. **Have Props Handy:** Some exercises may require props like a chair for balance, a towel for cushioning, or a strap for stretching. Keep these items within reach so you can easily incorporate them into your routine.

By following these guidelines, you can create a safe and comfortable practice area at home, enabling you to focus on your Wall Pilates exercises and achieve your fitness goals.

Essential Equipment Recommendations

To enhance your Wall Pilates experience and ensure a safe, effective workout, certain equipment can be incredibly useful. Here's a list of recommended items and their benefits:

1. **Yoga Mat:** A good-quality yoga mat provides cushioning and grip, making your exercises more comfortable and preventing slips. Look for mats with a non-slip surface and enough thickness to support your joints.

2. **Resistance Bands:** These are excellent for adding resistance to your exercises, helping to strengthen and tone muscles. They come in various levels of resistance, so you can choose the one that suits your fitness level. They're also lightweight and portable, making them easy to store.

3. **Yoga Blocks:** These can be used to provide support and stability in certain poses, making them more accessible and comfortable. They can also help with alignment and deepen your stretches.

4. **Stability Ball:** A stability ball can be used for a variety of exercises to improve balance, core strength, and flexibility. It's particularly useful for engaging the deep core muscles, which are crucial for overall stability.

5. **Chair:** A sturdy chair can be a valuable prop for balance and support during certain exercises, especially for those with mobility or balance issues. Ensure the chair is stable and doesn't have wheels.

6. **Towel:** A towel can be used for cushioning, support, and grip in various exercises. It's also handy for wiping away sweat during your workout.

7. **Ankle Weights:** For those looking to increase the intensity of leg exercises, ankle weights can add resistance and help strengthen the lower body.

8. **Foam Roller:** While not essential, a foam roller can be a great tool for self-massage and myofascial release, helping to relieve muscle tension and improve flexibility.

9. **Pilates Ring:** Also known as a magic circle, this tool can be used to add resistance to exercises, particularly for the inner and outer thighs, arms, and chest.

10. **Mirror:** Having a mirror in your practice area can be helpful for checking your form and ensuring that you're performing exercises correctly.

WALL PILATES FOR SENIORS TO LOSE WEIGHT

When choosing equipment, it's important to consider your individual needs and fitness level. Start with the basics, like a yoga mat and resistance bands, and gradually add more items as you become more comfortable with your practice. Always prioritize safety and comfort and consult with a healthcare professional or a qualified instructor if you're unsure about which equipment is right for you. With the right tools, you can enhance your Wall Pilates experience and enjoy a safe and effective workout from the comfort of your home.

Posture Check and Balance

Maintaining proper posture and balance is crucial in Wall Pilates, as it ensures the effectiveness of the exercises and prevents injuries. Here are some tips for seniors to stay aware of their posture and maintain balance:

1. **Start with a Posture Check:** Before beginning any exercise, stand against the wall with your heels, buttocks, shoulders, and head touching the wall. This position helps you feel what proper alignment feels like. Try to maintain this alignment throughout your exercises.

2. **Engage Your Core:** Your core muscles are key to maintaining balance and stability. Before starting an exercise, take a deep breath in, and as you exhale, gently draw your navel towards your spine. This engages your core and provides a strong foundation for your movements.

3. **Focus on Slow, Controlled Movements:** Rushing through exercises can lead to improper form. Move slowly and

deliberately, paying attention to each part of your body and how it aligns with the rest.

4. **Use Visual Cues:** If possible, practice in front of a mirror. This allows you to observe your posture and make adjustments in real time. Pay attention to whether your shoulders are level, your spine is straight, and your hips are aligned.

5. **Listen to Your Body:** Be mindful of how each movement feels. If something doesn't feel right, stop and readjust. Pain or discomfort is a sign that your posture might be off.

6. **Practice Balance Exercises:** Incorporate specific balance exercises into your routine, such as standing on one leg or using a balance pad. These exercises help improve your proprioception, or your body's ability to sense its position in space.

7. **Seek Feedback:** If you're unsure about your posture, consider working with a certified Pilates instructor or a physical therapist. They can provide personalized feedback and help you develop a better awareness of your body's alignment.

By regularly checking your posture and focusing on balance, you can enhance the effectiveness of your Wall Pilates practice and enjoy a safer, more beneficial workout.

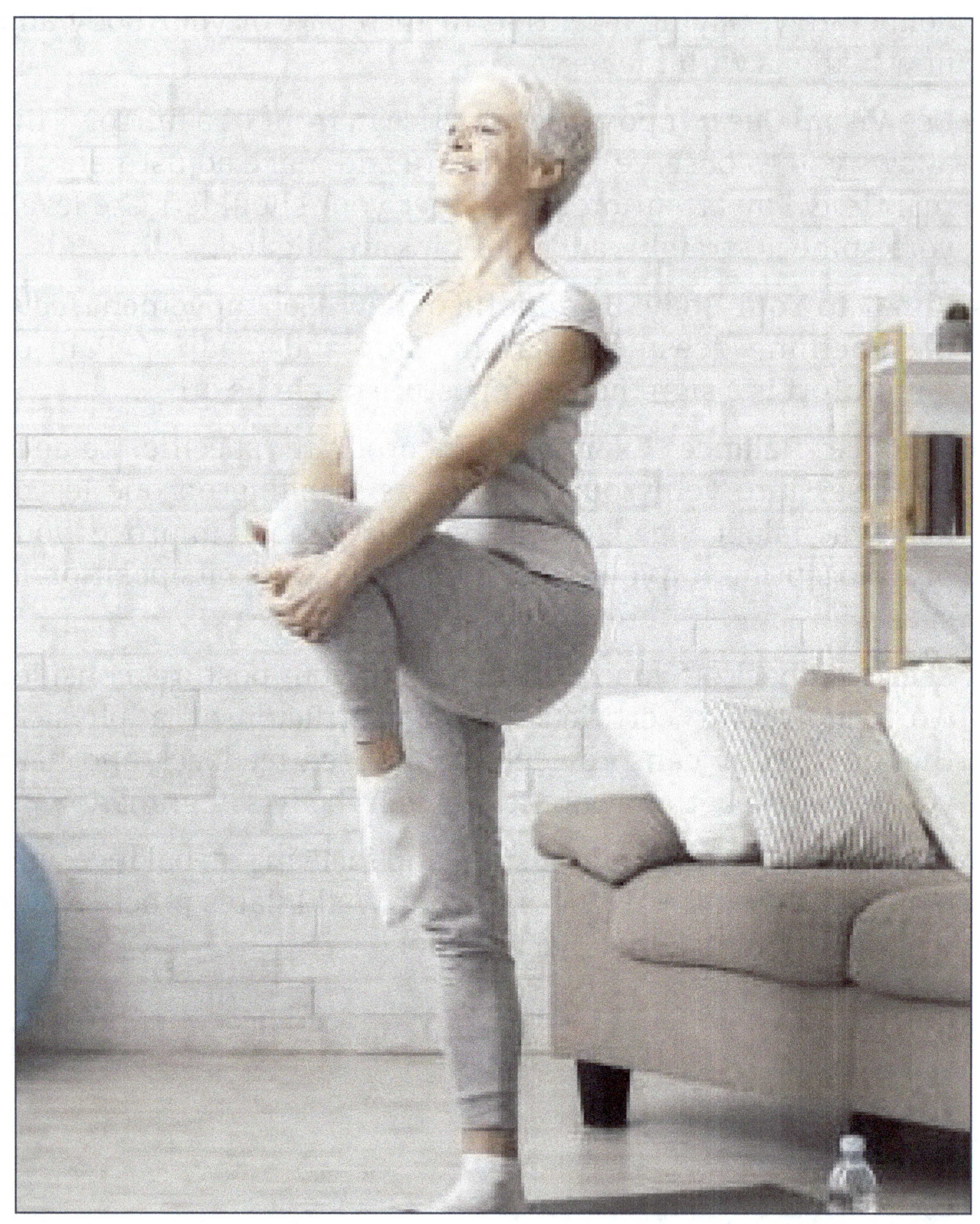

WALL PILATES FOR SENIORS TO LOSE WEIGHT

CORE AND BALANCE EXERCISES

Wall Heel Lifts

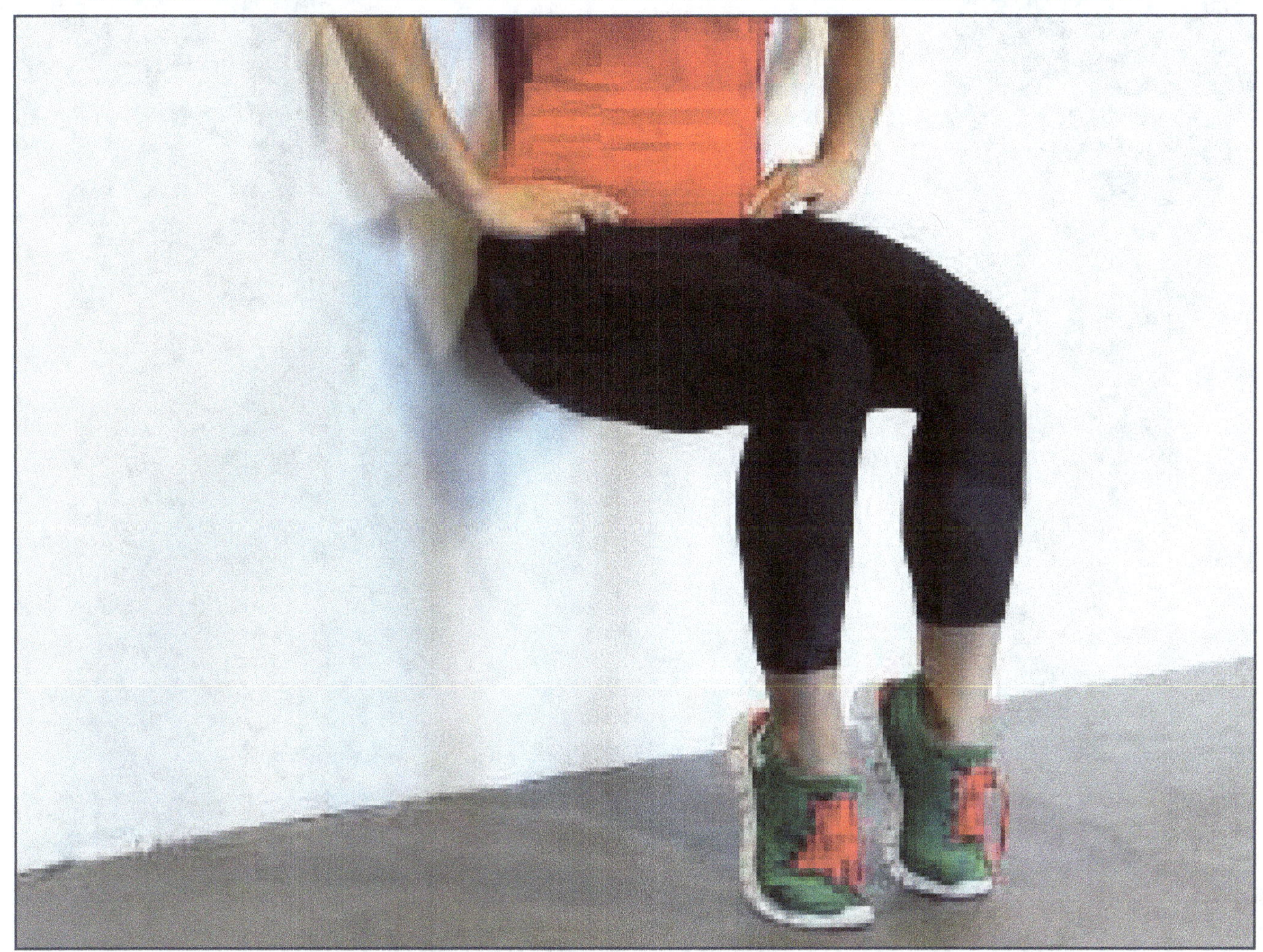

- Place your feet hip-width apart and lean your back against the wall.
- Press your lower back gently into the wall.
- Slowly lift your heels off the ground, rising onto your toes.
- After a little period of holding, bring your heels back down.
- Repeat 10-15 times, focusing on balance and control.

Wall Assisted Leg Balance

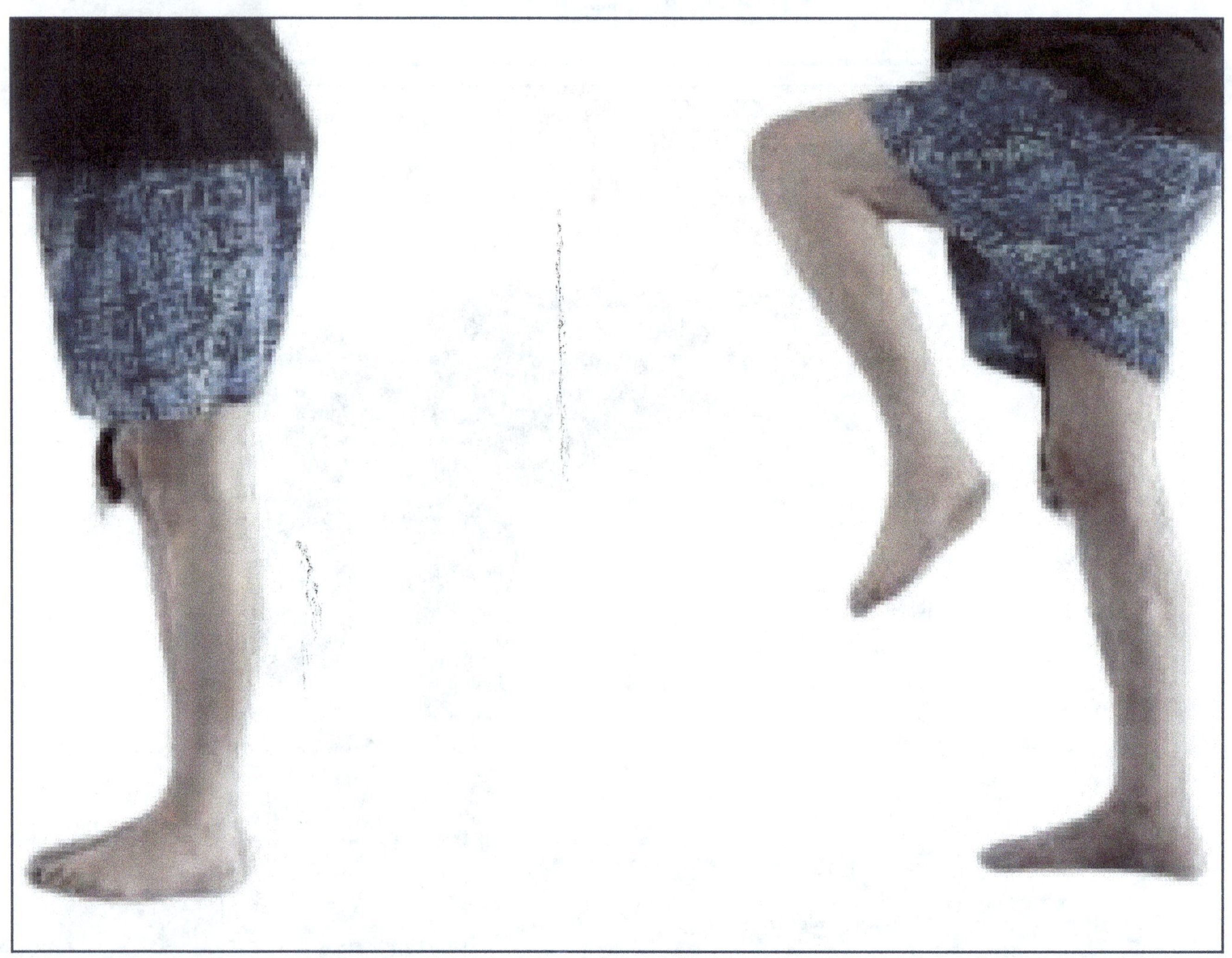

- Face the wall, standing arm's length away.
- For support, place your palms against the wall.
- Shift your weight onto your left foot.
- Slowly lift your right foot off the ground, keeping your leg straight.
- Hold the position for 5-10 seconds, then switch legs.
- Repeat 5-10 times on each leg, maintaining stability.

Pelvic Tilt

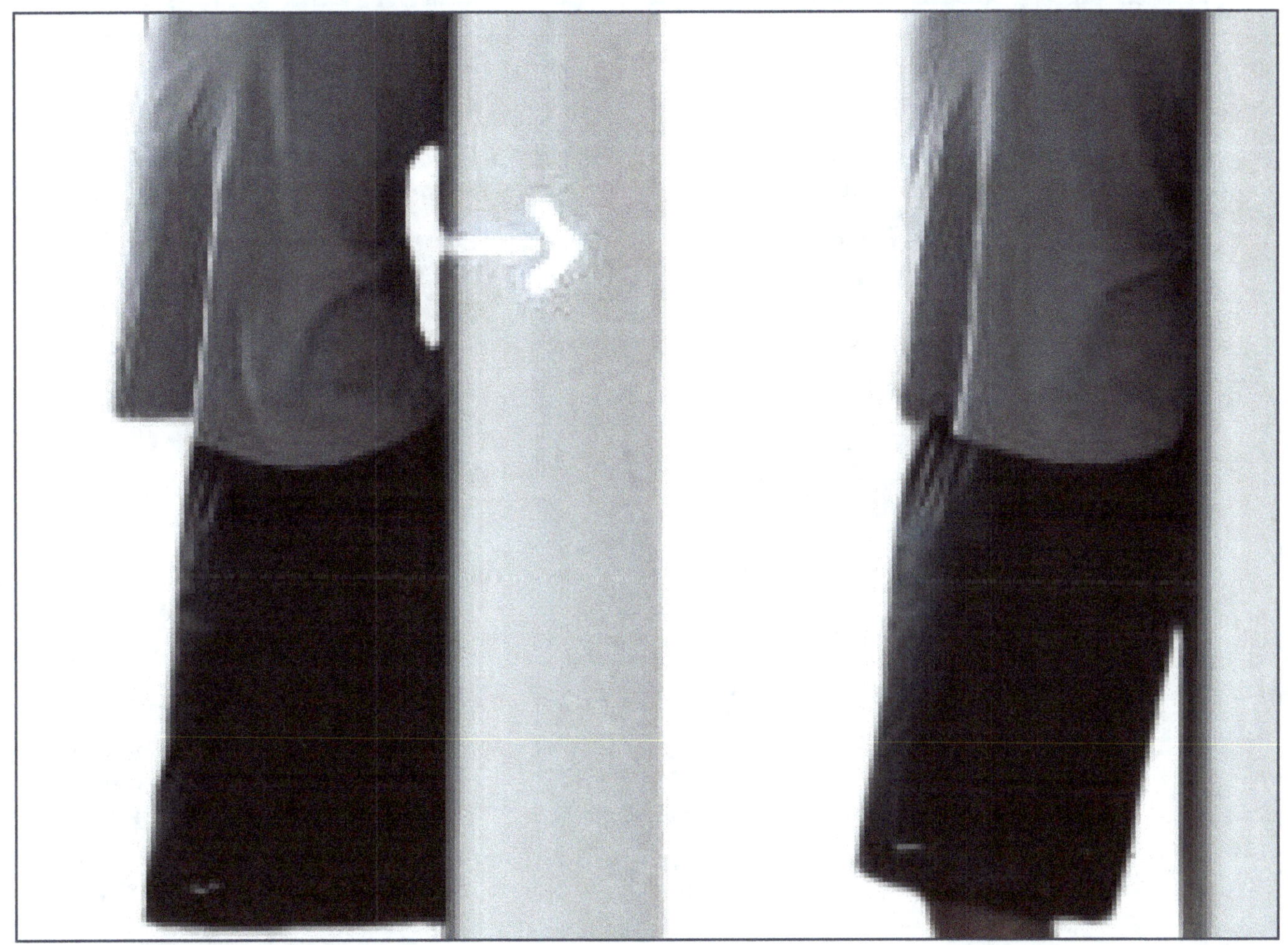

- Stand with your back against the wall, feet slightly forward.
- Flatten your lower back against the wall by tilting your pelvis upward.
- Hold for a few seconds, then release.
- Repeat ten to fifteen times, paying attention to activating your core muscles.

Wall Plank

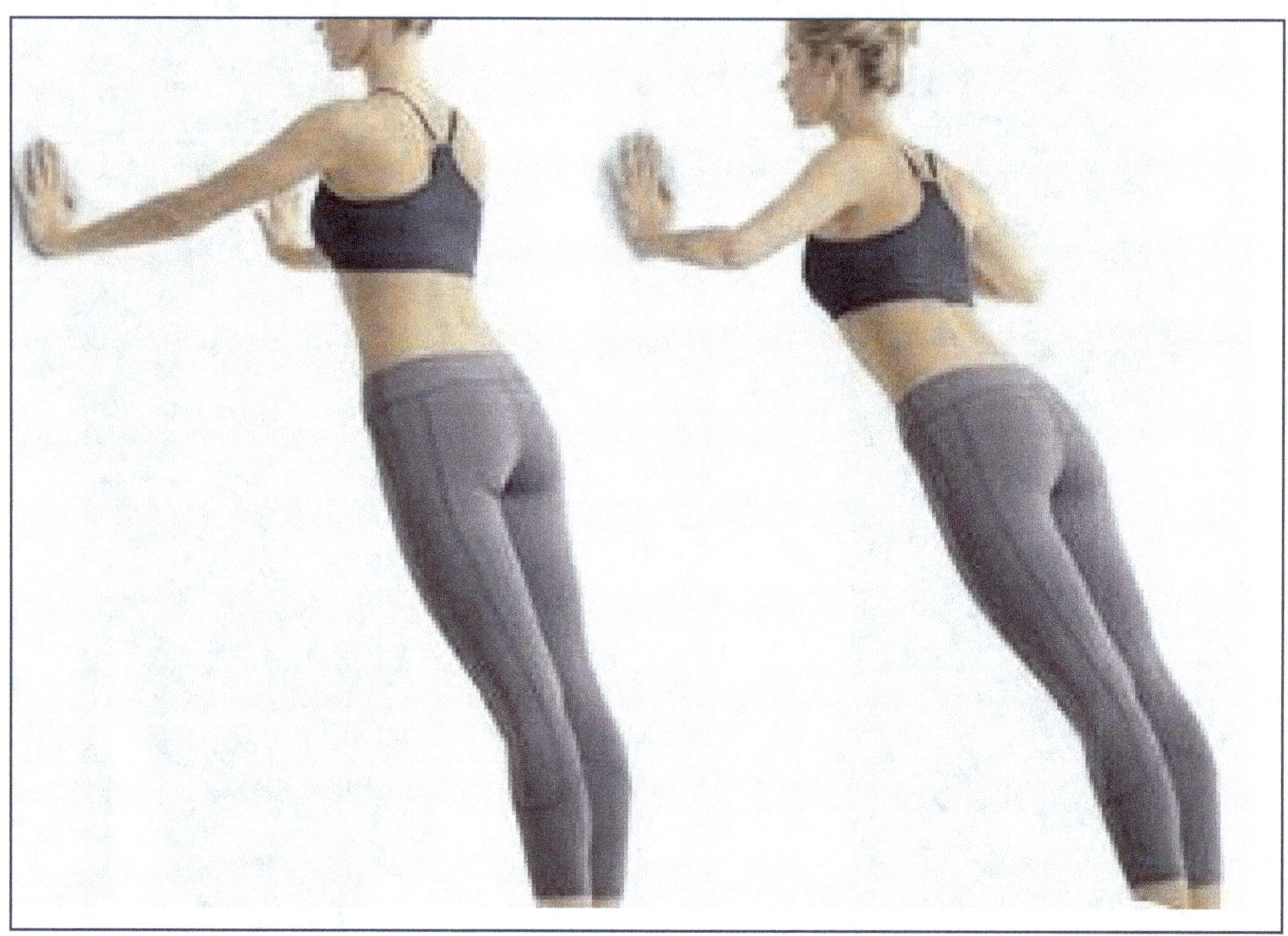

- Face the wall, standing arm's length away.
- Put your hands shoulder-height on the wall.
- Retrace your steps until your head to heels are in a straight line.
- Hold this position for 15-30 seconds, keeping your core engaged.
- Return to the starting position and repeat 2-3 times.

Wall Assisted Bridge

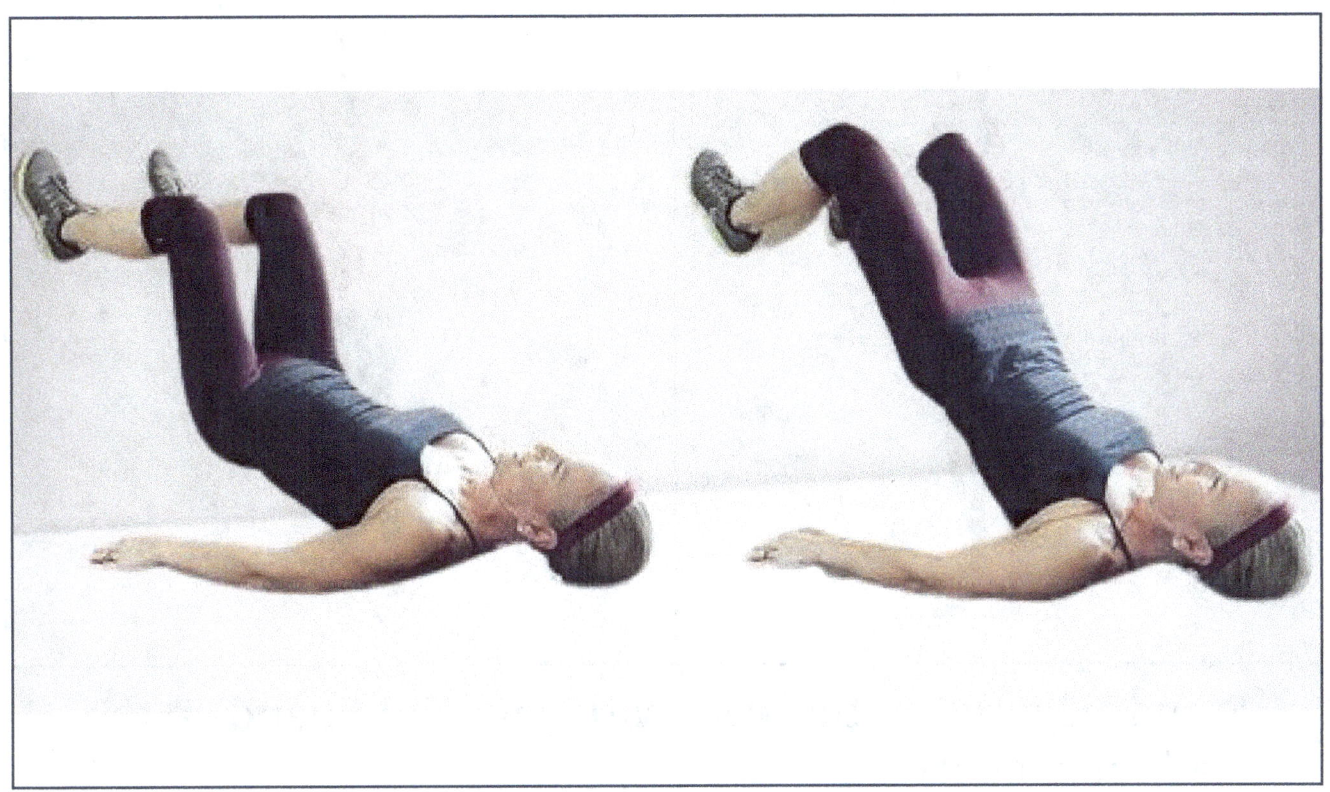

- Lie on your back with your feet flat on the ground, close to a wall.
- Place your feet on the wall, knees bent at a 90-degree angle.
- Press your feet into the wall and lift your hips towards the ceiling.
- Hold for a few seconds, then slowly lower your hips back down.
- Repeat 10-15 times, focusing on lifting with your glutes and hamstrings.

Pelvic Drop

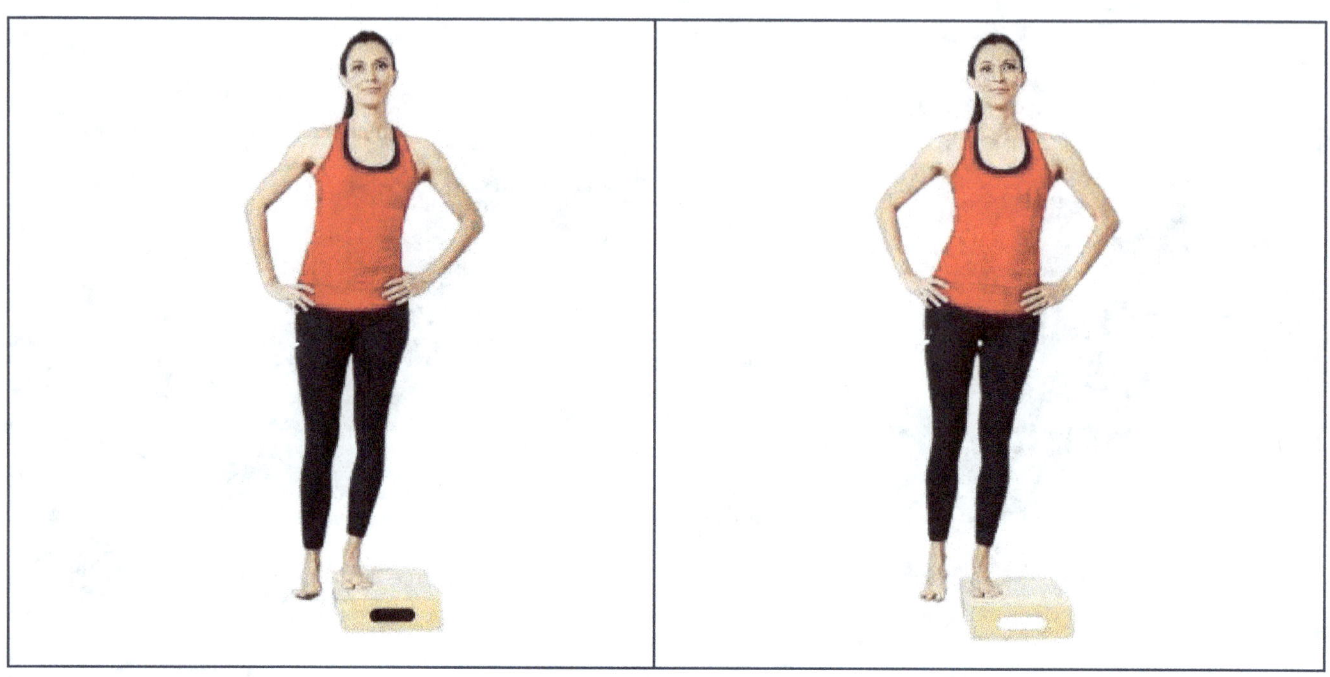

- Stand sideways to the wall, with your right hand on the wall for support.
- Lift your left leg slightly off the ground, keeping your hips level.
- Slowly lower your left hip without bending at the waist.
- Return your hips to their initial position.
- Repeat 10-15 times, then switch sides.
- Focus on controlled movements, using your core and hip muscles.

For each exercise, remember to breathe deeply and maintain good posture. Start with fewer repetitions and gradually increase as your strength and balance improve.

UPPER AND LOWER BODY EXERCISES

Arm Windows

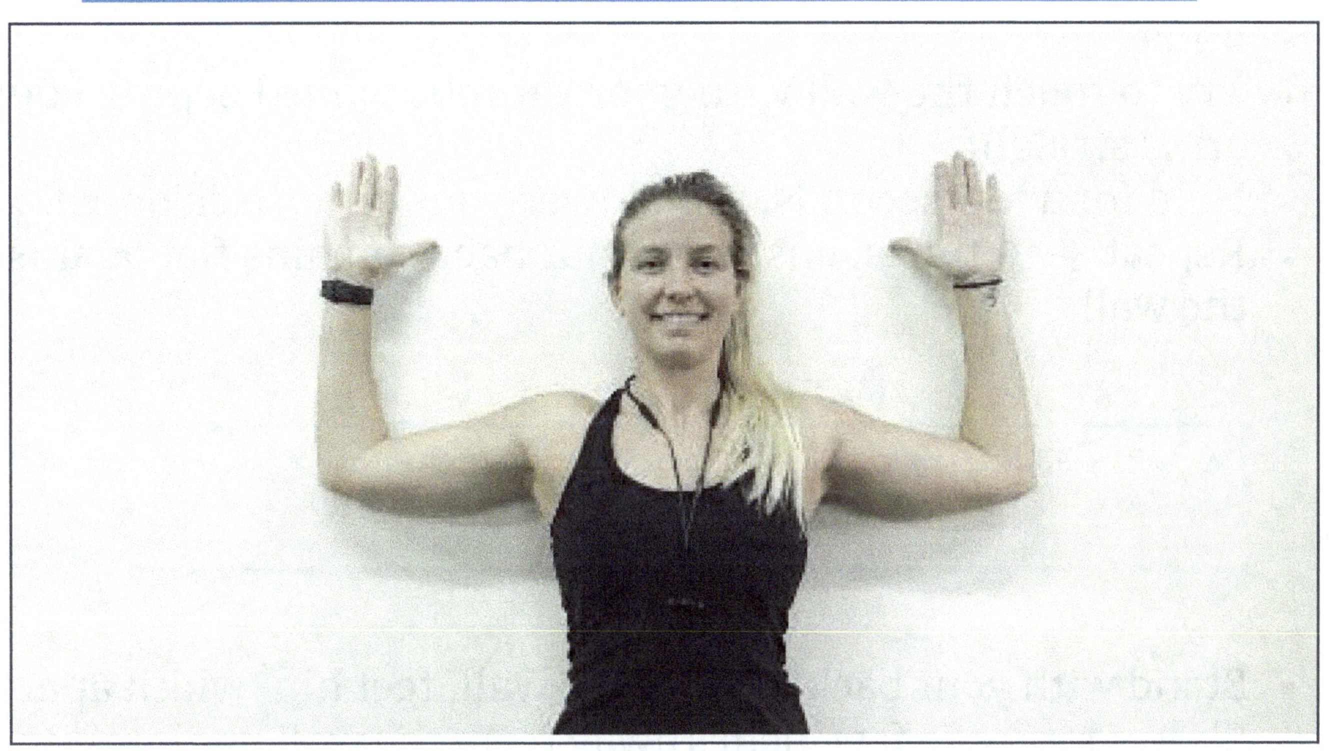

- Stand with your back against the wall, feet hip-width apart.
- Extend your arms out to the sides at shoulder height, palms facing forward.
- Bend your elbows to 90 degrees, keeping your upper arms parallel to the floor.
- Rotate your forearms up and back as if opening a window, then return to the starting position.
- Repeat 10-15 times, focusing on shoulder mobility.

Wall Arm Check

- Stand with your back against the wall, feet hip-width apart.
- Extend your arms straight up overhead, palms facing each other.
- Try to touch the wall with your thumbs while keeping your arms straight.
- Hold for a few seconds, then lower your arms back down.
- Repeat 5-10 times, ensuring your back remains flat against the wall.

Wall Little Leg Lifts

- Stand with your back against the wall, feet hip-width apart.
- Slide your feet a few inches away from the wall, maintaining contact with your upper back and hips.
- Lift one foot slightly off the ground, no more than a few inches.
- Hold for a few seconds, then switch to the other leg.
- Repeat 10-15 times on each leg, focusing on balance and stability.

Wall Push-Ups

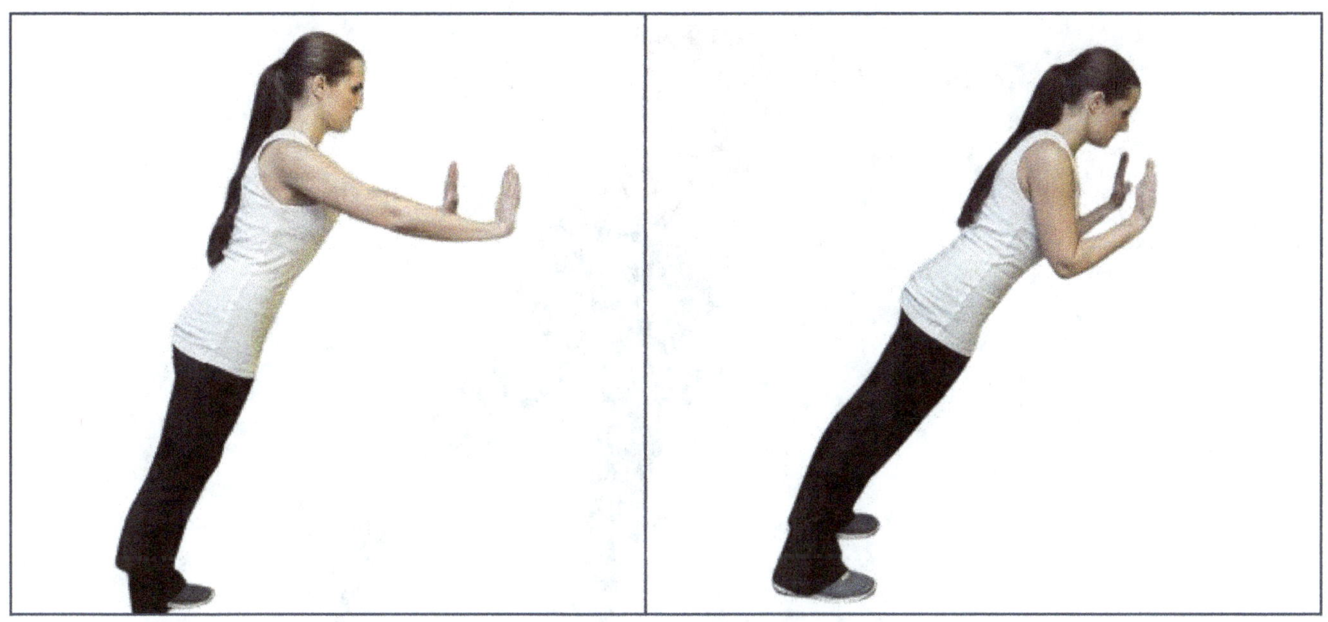

- Face the wall, standing arm's length away with feet hip-width apart.
- Place your palms on the wall at shoulder height.
- Bend your elbows and lean your body towards the wall, keeping your feet flat on the ground.
- Push back to the starting position, extending your arms fully.
- Repeat 10-15 times, maintaining a straight line from head to heels.

Wall Back Leg Lifts

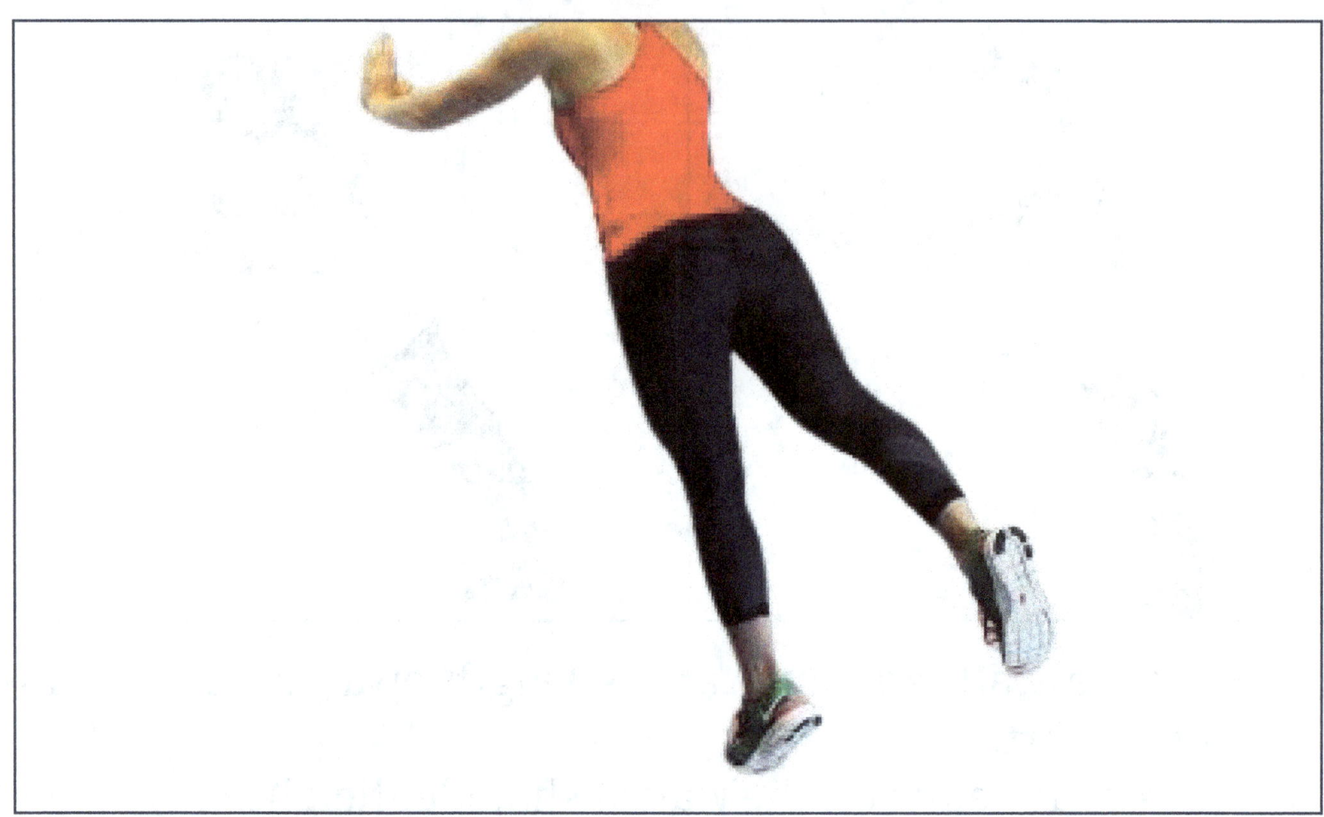

- Stand facing the wall, hands on the wall for support.
- Lift one leg straight behind you, keeping your hips square and back straight.
- Hold for a few seconds, then lower the leg back down.
- Repeat 10-15 times on each leg, engaging your glutes and hamstrings.

Wall Side Leg Lifts

- Stand sideways to the wall, with one hand on the wall for support.
- Lift the leg furthest from the wall out to the side, keeping your body upright.
- Hold for a few seconds, then lower the leg back down.
- Repeat 10-15 times on each leg, focusing on hip abductor strength.

Wall Calf Stretch

- Stand facing the wall, about an arm's length away.
- Place your hands on the wall at shoulder height.
- Step one foot back, keeping it straight, and press the heel into the floor.
- Bend your front knee slightly, keeping your back leg straight and heel on the ground.
- Hold the stretch for 20-30 seconds, then switch legs.
- Repeat 2-3 times on each leg, feeling the stretch in your calf muscles.

Wall Knee Bends

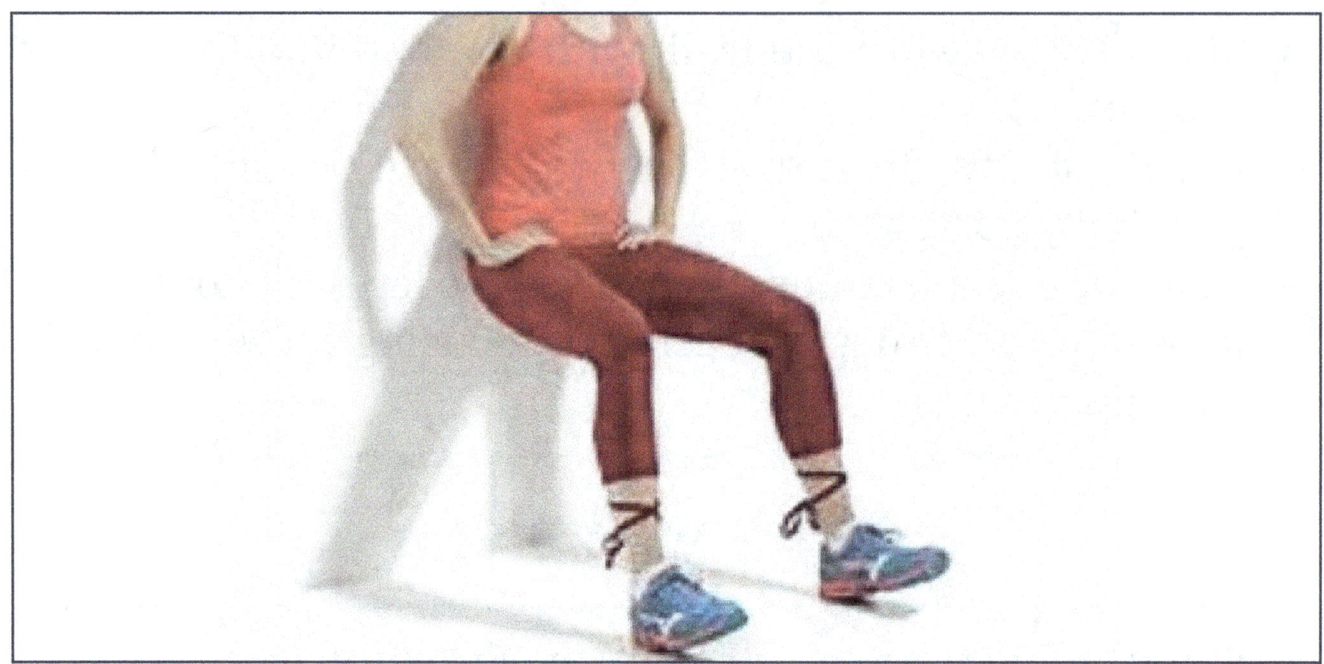

- Stand with your back against the wall, feet hip-width apart.

- Walk your feet out slightly, keeping your back flat against the wall.

- Slowly bend your knees, sliding down the wall until your knees are at a 90-degree angle.

- Hold for a few seconds, then straighten your legs to return to the starting position.

- Repeat 10-15 times, focusing on control and maintaining contact with the wall.

Wall Sidestep

- Stand with your side against the wall, feet together.
- Place your hand on the wall for balance.
- Step sideways with one foot, then bring the other foot to meet it.
- Take 10-15 steps in one direction, then switch and step in the opposite direction.
- Focus on smooth, controlled movements and maintaining an upright posture.

Wall Leg Extension

- Stand with your back against the wall, feet hip-width apart.
- Shift your weight to your left leg, keeping it slightly bent for stability.
- Lift your right foot off the ground and extend your right leg straight out in front of you, keeping your knee at hip height.
- Hold the extension for a few seconds, focusing on engaging your quadriceps (front thigh muscle).
- Slowly bend your knee and return your foot to the floor.
- Repeat 10-15 times on each leg, ensuring your back remains flat against the wall.

Wall Abdominal Crunches

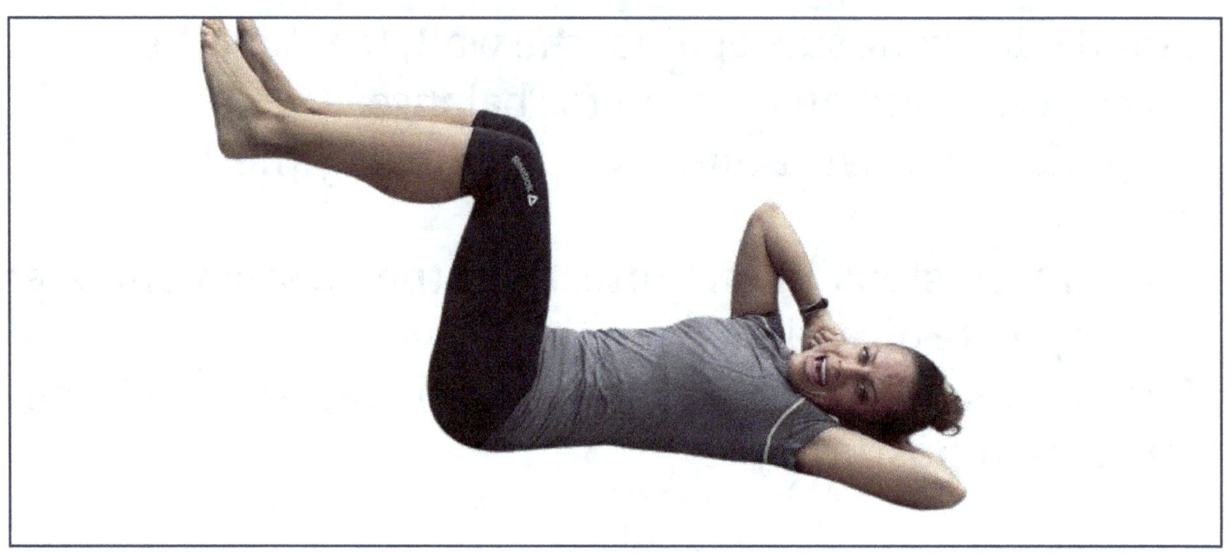

- Lie on your back on the floor, with your legs bent and feet flat against the wall. Your knees should be at a 90-degree angle.
- Place your hands behind your head or across your chest.
- Engage your core muscles and lift your upper body toward your knees, keeping your lower back pressed into the floor.
- Hold the crunch position for a few seconds, then slowly lower your upper body back to the floor.
- Repeat 10-15 times, focusing on using your abdominal muscles to lift and lower your torso.

For both exercises, maintain a steady breathing pattern and focus on controlled movements. Adjust the number of repetitions based on your fitness level and comfort.

FLEXIBILITY AND MOBILITY EXERCISES

Neck Stretch

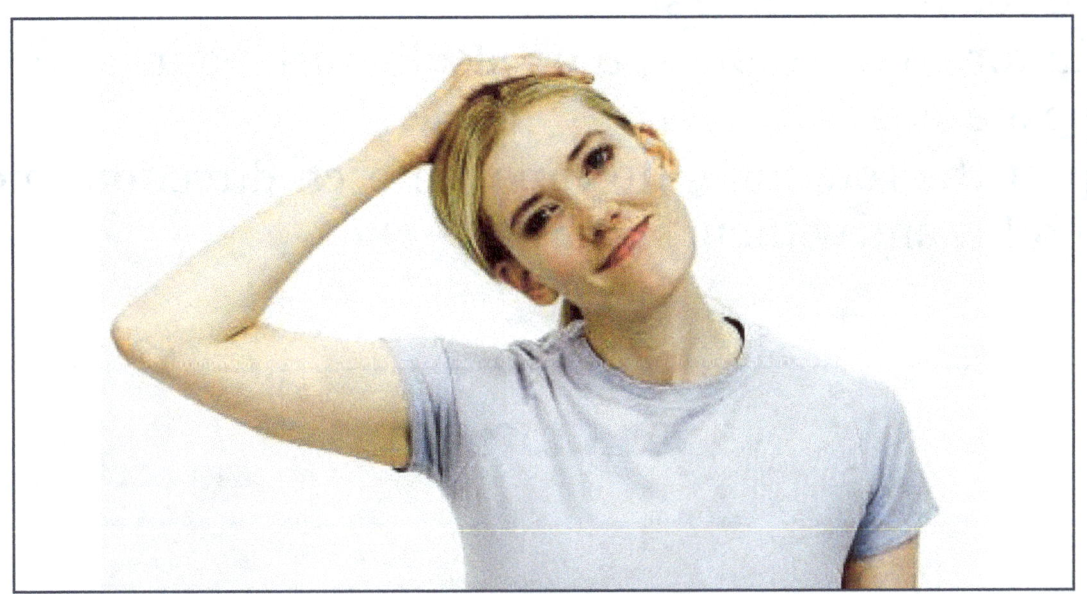

- Sit or stand with your back straight and shoulders relaxed.
- Gently tilt your head to one side, bringing your ear toward your shoulder, until you feel a stretch on the opposite side of your neck.
- Hold the stretch for 20-30 seconds, then slowly return to the starting position.
- Repeat on the other side.
- Avoid shrugging your shoulder or twisting your neck during the stretch.

Neck Rotations

- Sit or stand with your back straight and shoulders relaxed.
- Slowly turn your head to one side, keeping your chin level, until you feel a gentle stretch.
- Hold for a few seconds, then slowly turn your head to the opposite side.
- Repeat the rotation 5-10 times in each direction, moving smoothly and without straining.

Arm Lifts

- Stand or sit with your back straight and arms at your sides.
- Slowly raise your arms out to the sides and up overhead, keeping them straight.
- Hold for a moment when your arms are fully extended above your head, then slowly lower them back to your sides.
- Repeat 10-15 times, focusing on smooth, controlled movements.

Knee Lifts

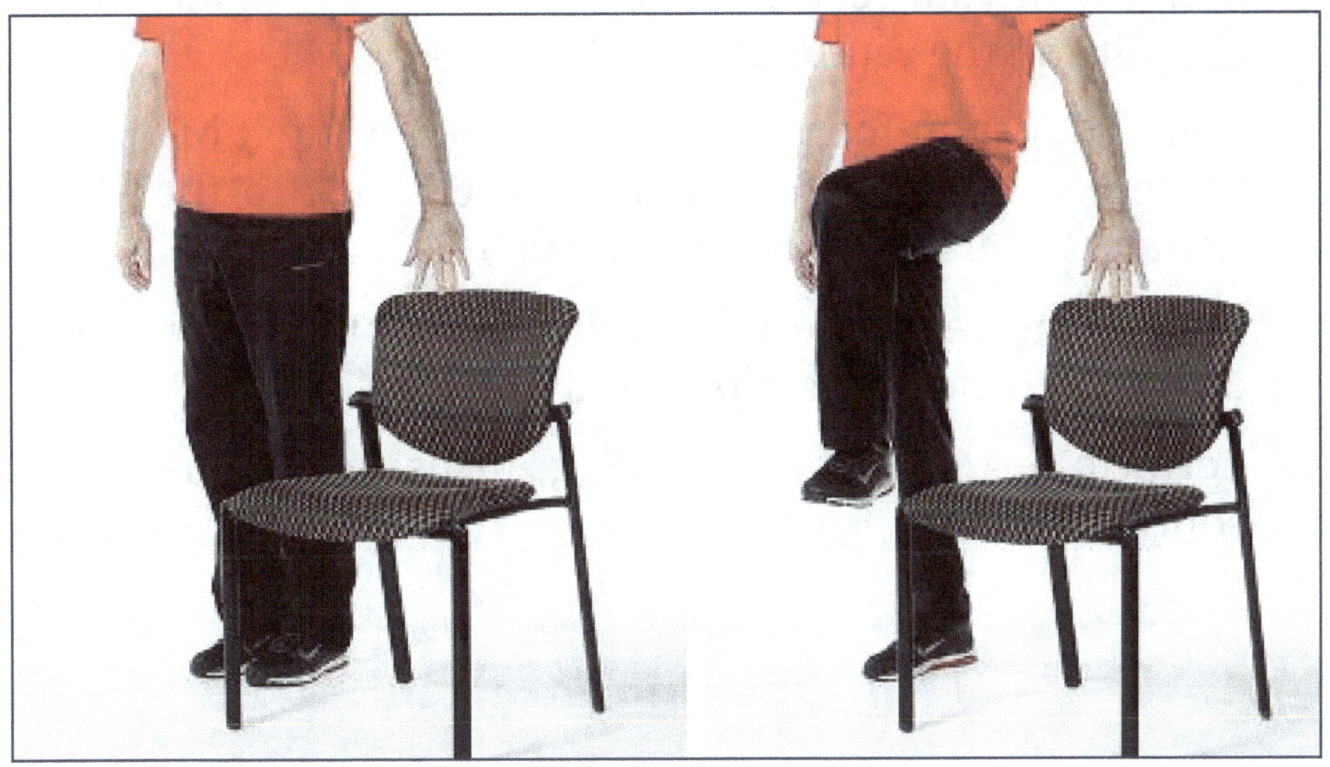

- Stand with your feet hip-width apart and hold onto a chair or wall for balance if needed.
- Slowly lift one knee toward your chest, keeping your back straight and the other leg slightly bent for stability.
- Hold for a few seconds, then lower your foot back to the ground.
- Repeat 10-15 times on each leg, focusing on engaging your core muscles.

Clock Exercises

- Stand with your feet hip-width apart and imagine you are standing in the center of a clock.

- Point your right foot to 12 o'clock, then bring it back to the center. Next, point to 3 o'clock, then back to the center. Continue pointing to 6 o'clock and 9 o'clock.

- Repeat the sequence with your left foot, pointing to 12 o'clock, 9 o'clock, 6 o'clock, and 3 o'clock.

- Perform 2-3 rounds on each leg, focusing on balance and control.

Hip Opening Stretch

- Sit on a chair with your feet flat on the ground and your back straight.
- Place your right ankle on your left knee, forming a figure-four shape.
- Gently press down on your right knee to increase the stretch in your right hip.
- Hold for 20-30 seconds, then switch legs and repeat.
- Do 2-3 repetitions on each side, focusing on opening the hips.

Arm Reach

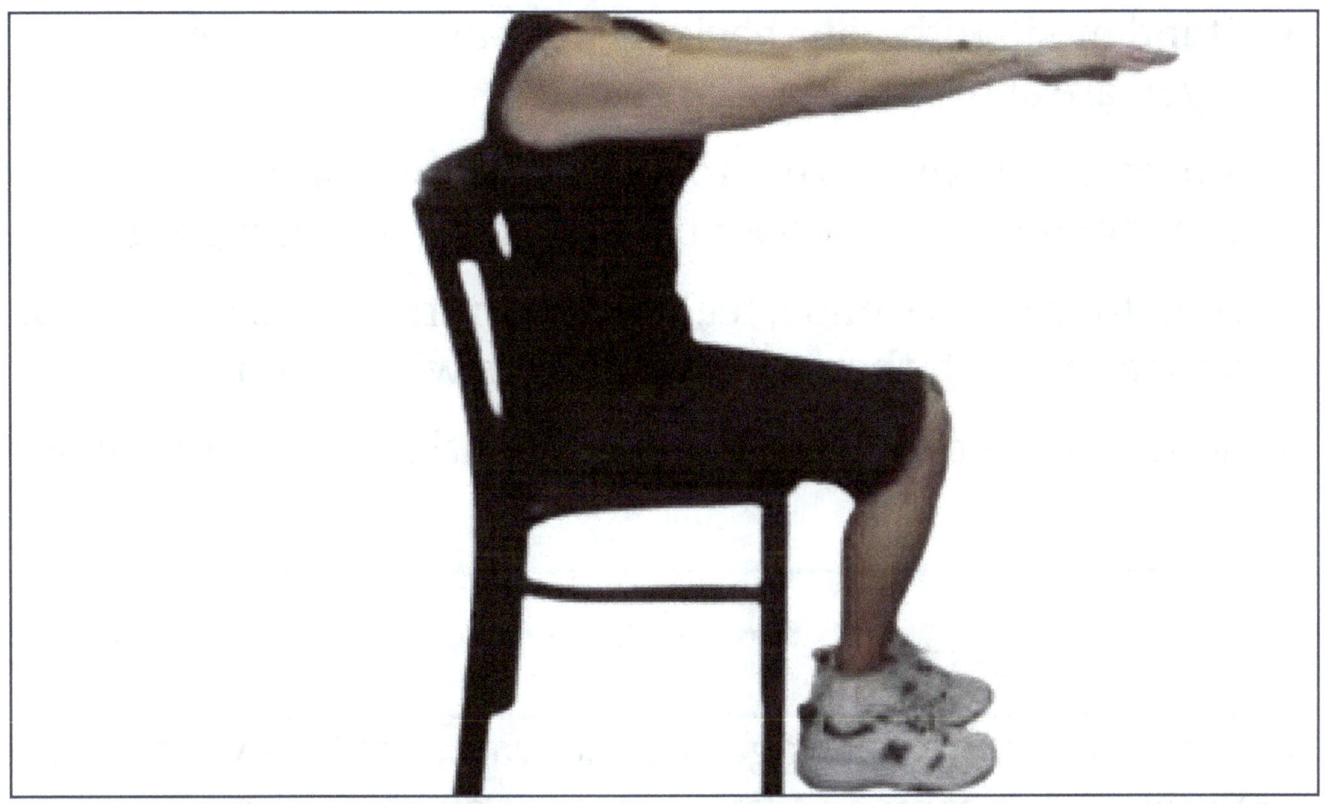

- Stand or sit with your back straight and arms at your sides.

- Reach one arm straight out in front of you, parallel to the ground.

- Hold for a few seconds, then slowly lower your arm back to your side.

- Repeat 10-15 times on each arm, focusing on extending fully without straining.

Hug a Tree

- Stand or sit with your back straight and arms open wide, as if you are about to hug a large tree.
- Slowly bring your arms together in front of you, rounding your shoulders and upper back slightly, as if hugging a tree.
- Hold for a few seconds, feeling the stretch across your upper back and chest, then open your arms wide again.
- Repeat 10-15 times, focusing on a gentle stretch and release.

Core Turn

- Stand with your back against the wall, feet hip-width apart.
- Extend your arms in front of you at shoulder height, palms facing each other.
- Keeping your hips and feet facing forward, gently rotate your torso to one side, leading with your arms.
- Hold for a few seconds, feeling the stretch in your core and back.
- Return to the center and repeat on the other side.
- Do 10-15 repetitions on each side, focusing on controlled movements.

Hip Opening Stretch

- Sit on a chair with your feet flat on the ground and your back straight.
- Place your right ankle on your left knee, forming a figure-four shape.
- Gently press down on your right knee to increase the stretch in your right hip.
- Hold for 20-30 seconds, then switch legs and repeat.
- Do 2-3 repetitions on each side, focusing on opening the hips.

Single Leg Balance

- Stand near a wall or chair for support if needed.
- Shift your weight onto one leg, keeping a slight bend in the knee.
- Lift your other foot off the ground and hold the position for 10-20 seconds.
- Switch legs and repeat.
- Do 5-10 repetitions on each leg, focusing on balance and stability.

Wall Calf Raises

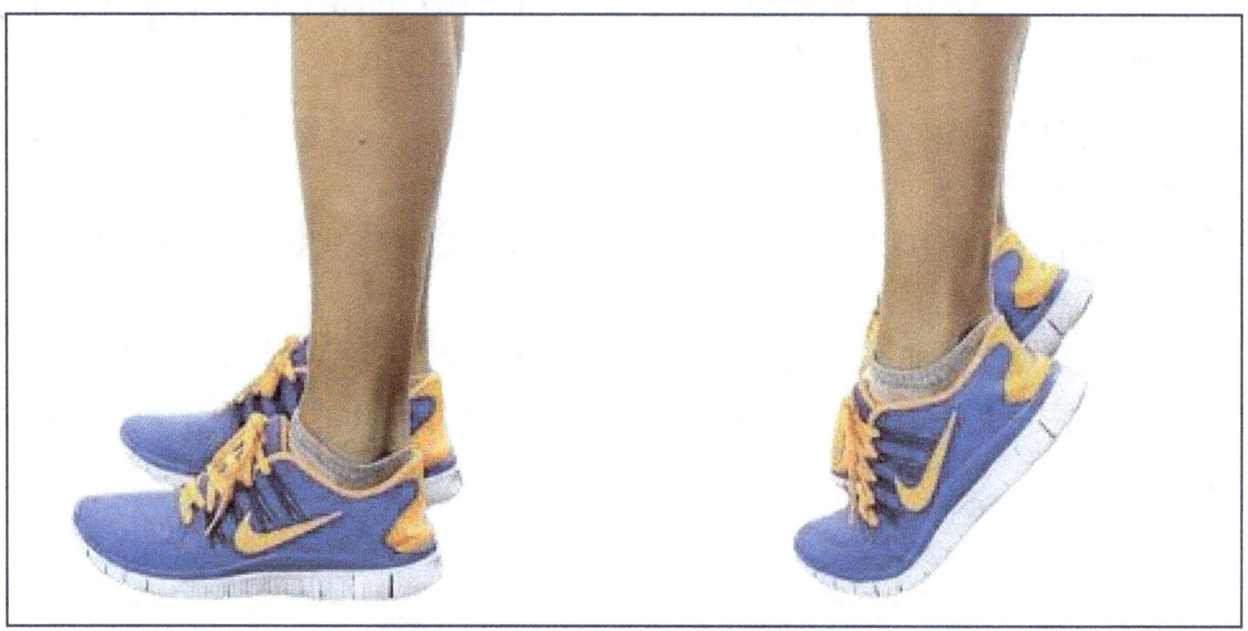

- Stand facing a wall with your feet hip-width apart.
- Place your hands on the wall for support.
- Slowly raise your heels off the ground, coming onto your toes.
- Hold for a few seconds, then slowly lower your heels back to the ground.
- Do 10-15 repetitions, focusing on strengthening your calf muscles.

For each exercise, maintain good posture and adjust the intensity and repetitions according to your comfort and fitness level.

NUTRITIONAL GUIDE FOR WALL PILATES PRACTITIONERS

Basic Nutrition Principles

For seniors practicing Wall Pilates for effective weight loss, understanding basic nutrition principles is crucial. Here are key guidelines:

Balanced Diet: Emphasize a balanced diet that includes a variety of foods from all food groups: fruits, vegetables, whole grains, lean proteins, and healthy fats. This ensures you get a wide range of nutrients essential for overall health and energy.

Portion Control: Be mindful of portion sizes to avoid overeating. Using smaller plates and measuring servings can help manage portions, keeping calorie intake in check.

Hydration: Stay well-hydrated by drinking plenty of water throughout the day. Adequate hydration is important for digestion, energy levels, and overall well-being.

Protein Intake: Include adequate protein in your diet to support muscle repair and growth, especially important for seniors engaging in exercise like Wall Pilates. Lean sources of protein such as chicken, fish, tofu, legumes, and low-fat dairy products are recommended.

Healthy Fats: Incorporate healthy fats into your diet, such as those found in avocados, nuts, seeds, and olive oil. These fats are essential for heart health and can help keep you feeling full and satisfied.

Limit Added Sugars: Reduce the intake of added sugars found in sweets, sugary drinks, and processed foods. Instead, opt for natural sources of sweetness like fruits.

Fiber-Rich Foods: Include fiber-rich foods like whole grains, fruits, vegetables, and legumes in your meals. Fiber aids in digestion, helps control blood sugar levels, and can contribute to a feeling of fullness, aiding in weight management.

Regular Meals: Eat regular meals and snacks to keep your metabolism steady and energy levels consistent. Skipping meals can lead to overeating later and may impact your performance during Wall Pilates sessions.

By adhering to these basic nutrition principles, seniors practicing Wall Pilates can support their weight loss goals while maintaining a healthy and balanced diet.

Foods to Fuel Your Wall Pilates Practice

Quinoa and Black Bean Salad

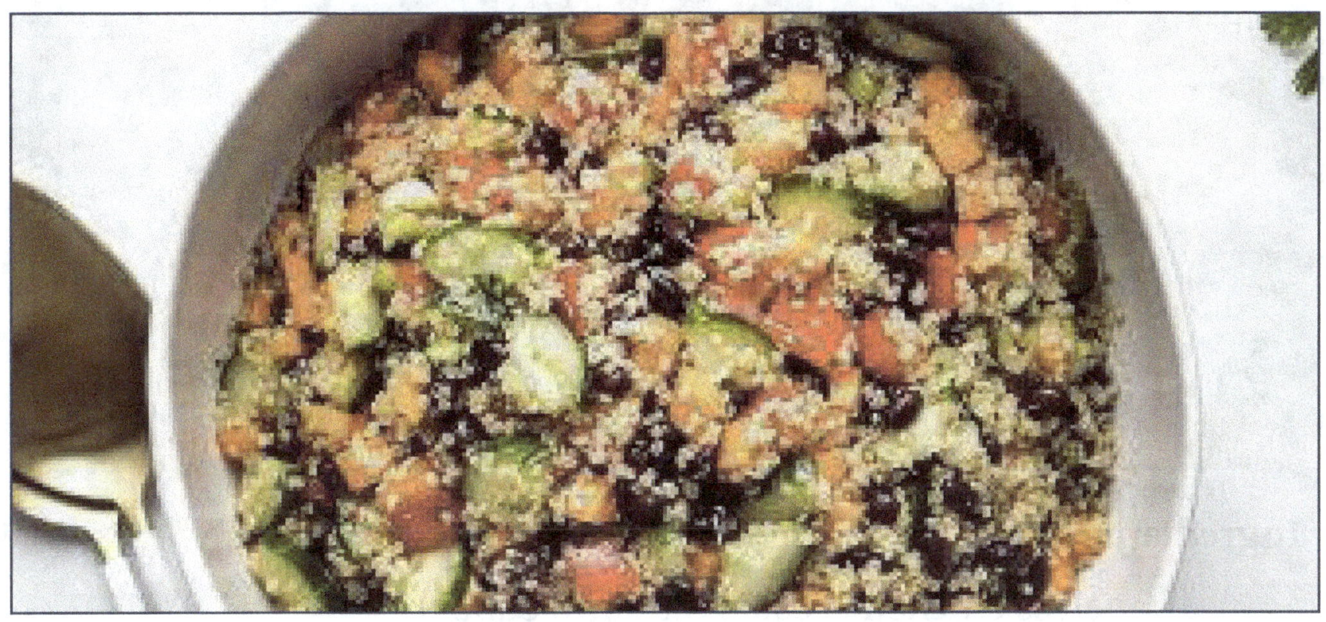

Ingredients:

- 1 cup cooked quinoa
- 1 cup black beans (drained and rinsed)
- 1 diced red bell pepper
- 1/4 cup chopped cilantro.
- 2 tbsp lime juice
- 1 tbsp olive oil, salt, and pepper.

Instructions:

In a bowl, mix quinoa, black beans, red bell pepper, and cilantro. In a separate bowl, whisk together lime juice, olive oil, salt, and pepper. Pour the dressing over the salad and toss to combine.

Grilled Chicken and Vegetable Skewers

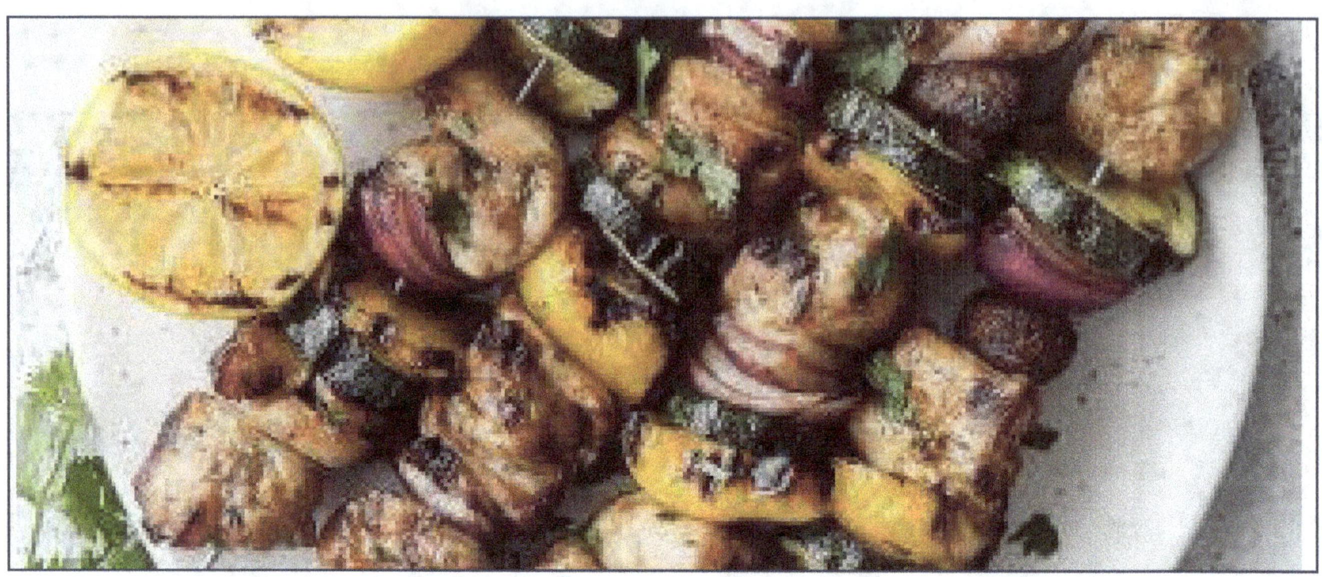

Ingredients:

- 2 boneless chicken breasts (cut into cubes)
- 1 zucchini (sliced)
- 1 red bell pepper (cut into squares)
- 1 onion (cut into squares)
- 2 tbsp olive oil
- 1 tbsp lemon juice, salt, and pepper.

Instructions:

Thread chicken, zucchini, bell pepper, and onion onto skewers. In a bowl, mix olive oil, lemon juice, salt, and pepper. Brush the mixture onto the skewers. Grill for 10-15 minutes, turning occasionally, until the chicken is cooked through.

Spinach and Feta Stuffed Chicken

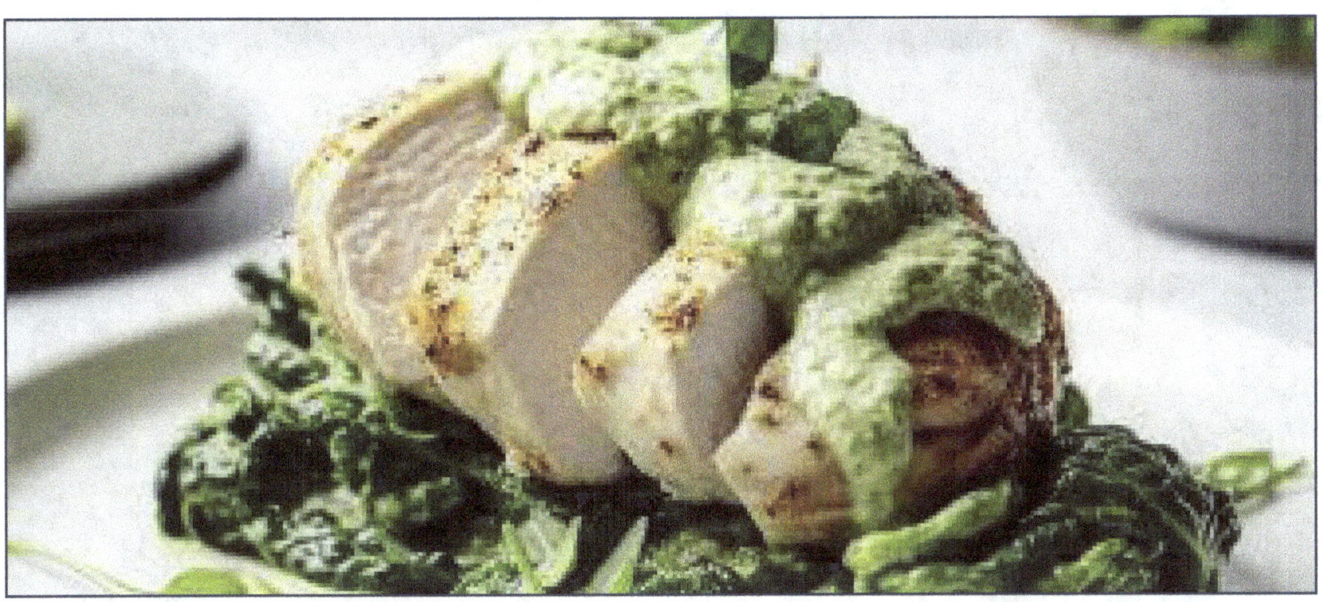

Ingredients:

- 2 boneless chicken breasts
- 1 cup fresh spinach
- 1/4 cup crumbled feta cheese.
- 1 clove garlic (minced)
- 1 tbsp olive oil, salt, and pepper.

Instructions:

Preheat oven to 375°F. Cut a pocket into each chicken breast. In a bowl, mix spinach, feta, garlic, salt, and pepper. Stuff the mixture into the chicken pockets. Secure with toothpicks. Heat olive oil in a pan and sear chicken on both sides. Transfer to the oven and bake for 20-25 minutes.

Lentil Soup

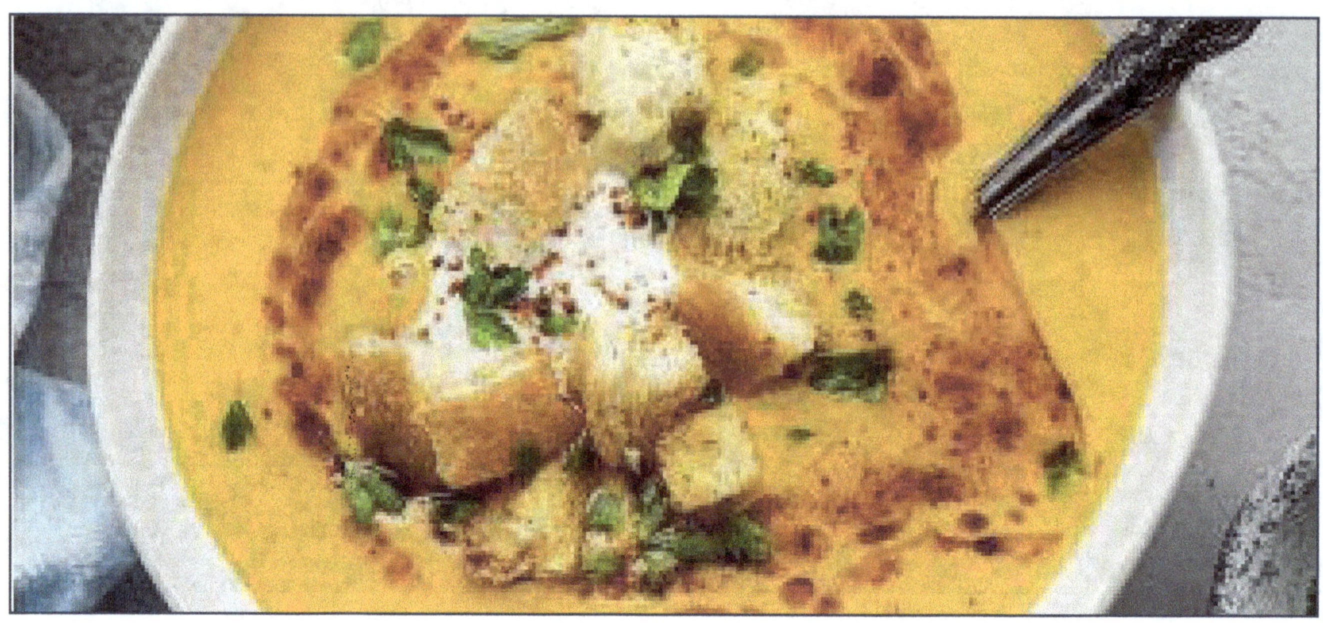

Ingredients:

- 1 cup lentils
- 1 diced onion
- 2 diced carrots
- 2 diced celery stalks
- 2 cloves garlic (minced)
- 4 cups vegetable broth
- 1 tsp cumin
- 1 tsp turmeric, salt, and pepper.

Instructions:

In a pot, sauté onion, carrots, celery, and garlic until softened. Add lentils, vegetable broth, cumin, turmeric, salt, and pepper. Bring to a boil, then reduce heat and simmer for 25-30 minutes.

Baked Salmon with Asparagus:

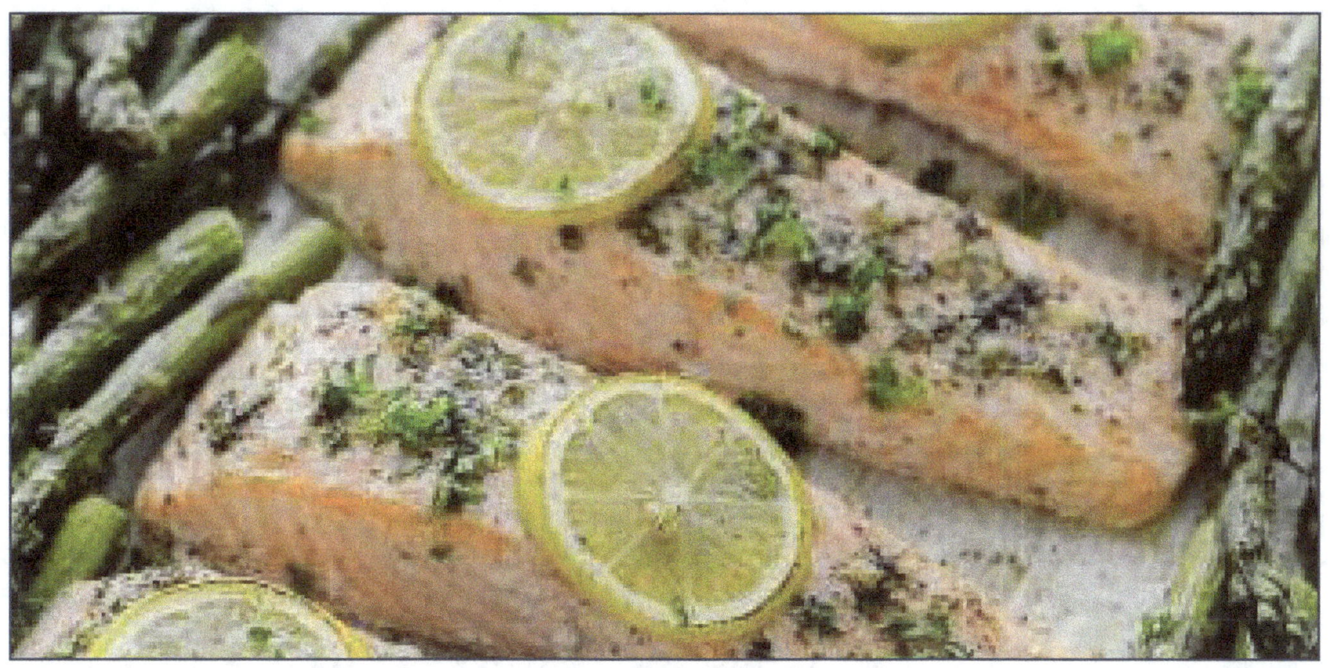

Ingredients:

- 2 salmon fillets
- 1 bunch asparagus (trimmed)
- 2 tbsp olive oil
- 1 lemon (sliced), salt, and pepper.

Instructions:

Preheat oven to 400°F. Place salmon and asparagus on a baking sheet. Drizzle with olive oil and season with salt and pepper. Top with lemon slices. Bake for 15-20 minutes.

Greek Yogurt Parfait

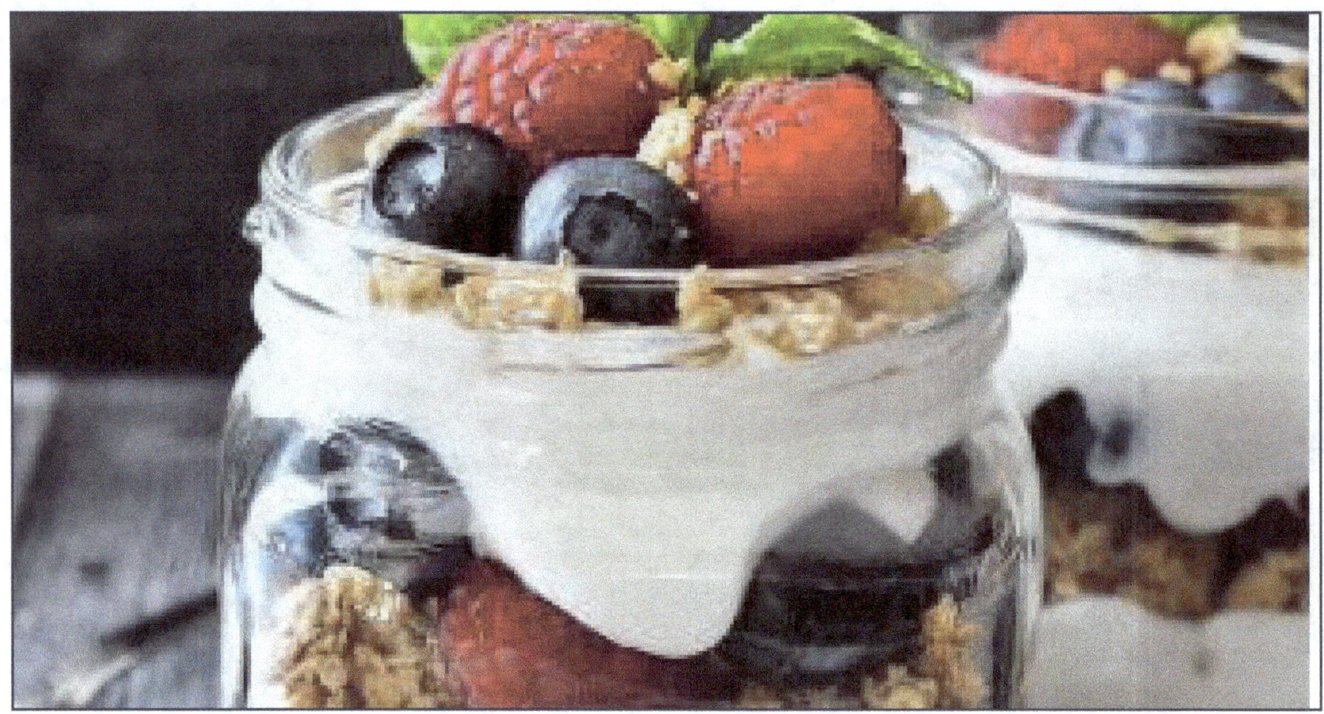

Ingredients:

- 1 cup Greek yogurt
- 1/2 cup mixed berries
- 1/4 cup granola
- 1 tbsp honey.

Instructions:

Layer Greek yogurt, mixed berries, and granola in a glass. Drizzle with honey.

Avocado and Egg Toast

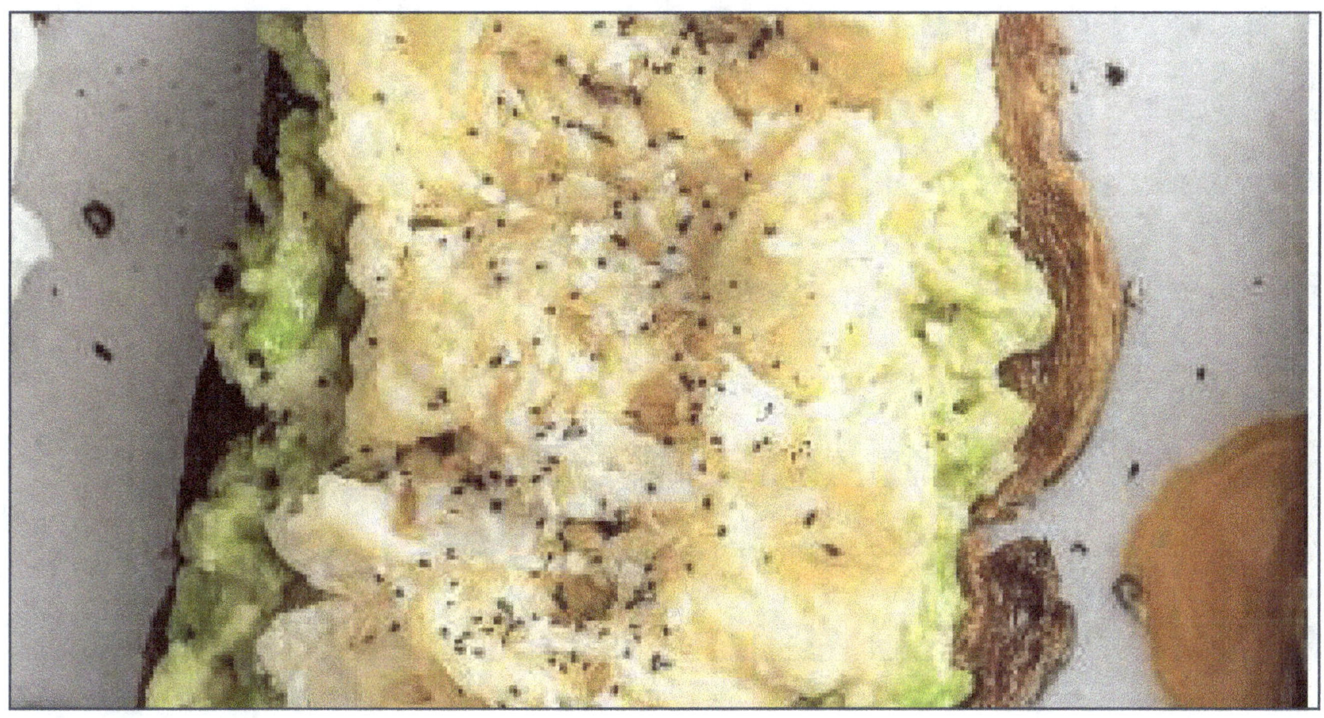

Ingredients:

- 1 slice whole-grain bread (toasted)
- 1/2 avocado (mashed)
- 1 poached egg, salt, and pepper.

Instructions:

Spread mashed avocado on toast. Top with a poached egg. Season with salt and pepper.

Turkey and Vegetable Stir-Fry

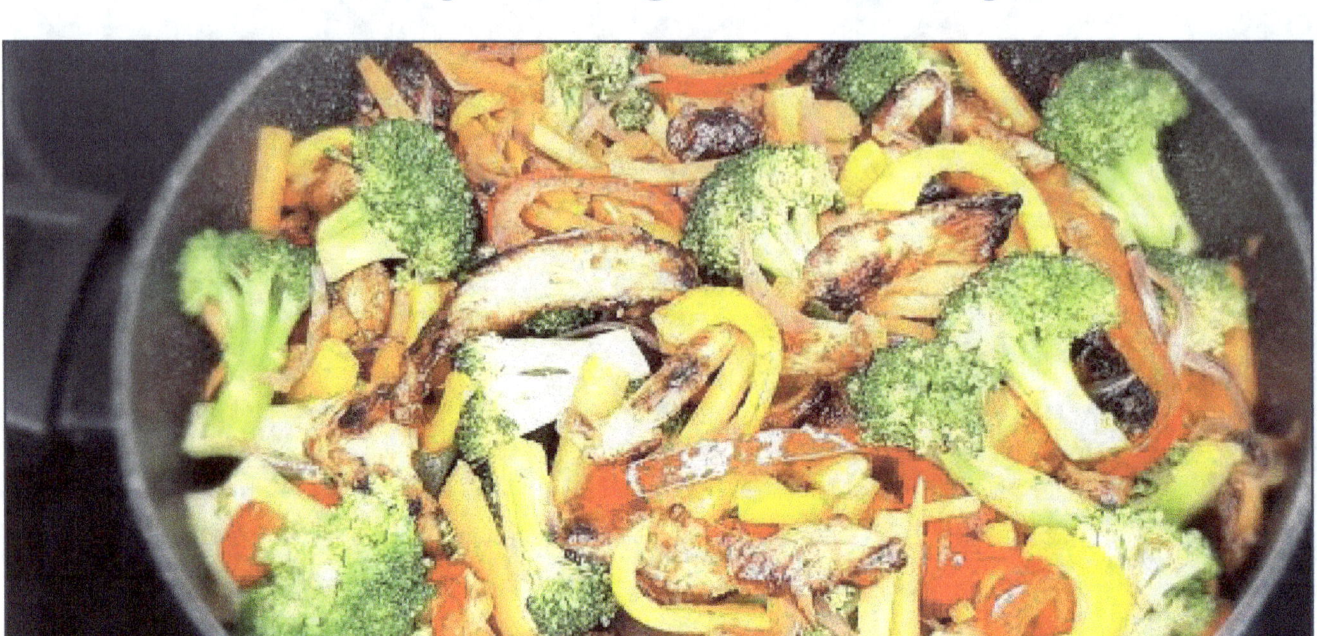

Ingredients:

- 1 lb ground turkey
- 2 cups mixed vegetables (e.g., bell peppers, broccoli, carrots)
- 2 tbsp soy sauce
- 1 tbsp olive oil
- 1 clove garlic (minced), salt, and pepper.

Instructions:

Heat olive oil in a pan. Add garlic and ground turkey. Cook until browned. Add vegetables and soy sauce. Stir-fry until vegetables are tender.

Cucumber and Tomato Salad

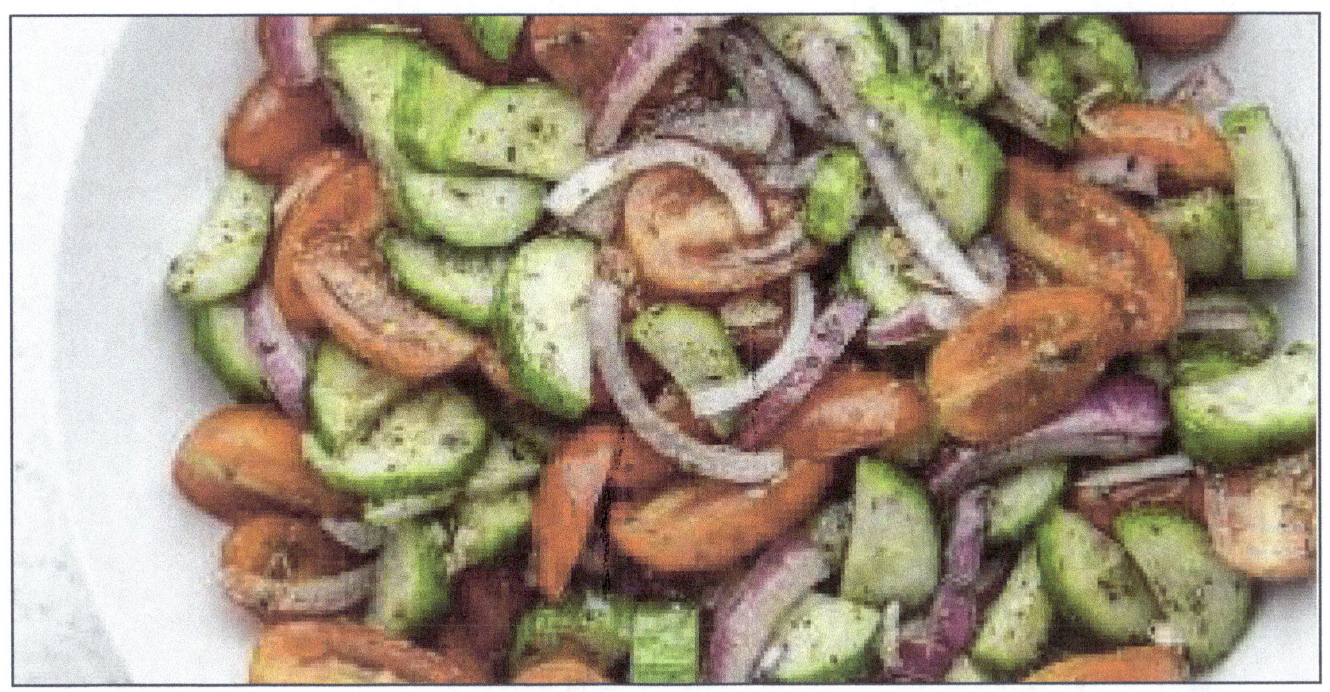

Ingredients:

- 1 cucumber (sliced)
- 2 tomatoes (chopped)
- 1/4 red onion (thinly sliced)
- 2 tbsp olive oil
- 1 tbsp vinegar, salt, and pepper.

Instructions:

In a bowl, mix cucumber, tomatoes, and red onion. In a separate bowl, whisk together olive oil, vinegar, salt, and pepper. Pour the dressing over the salad and toss to combine.

Mixed Berry Smoothie

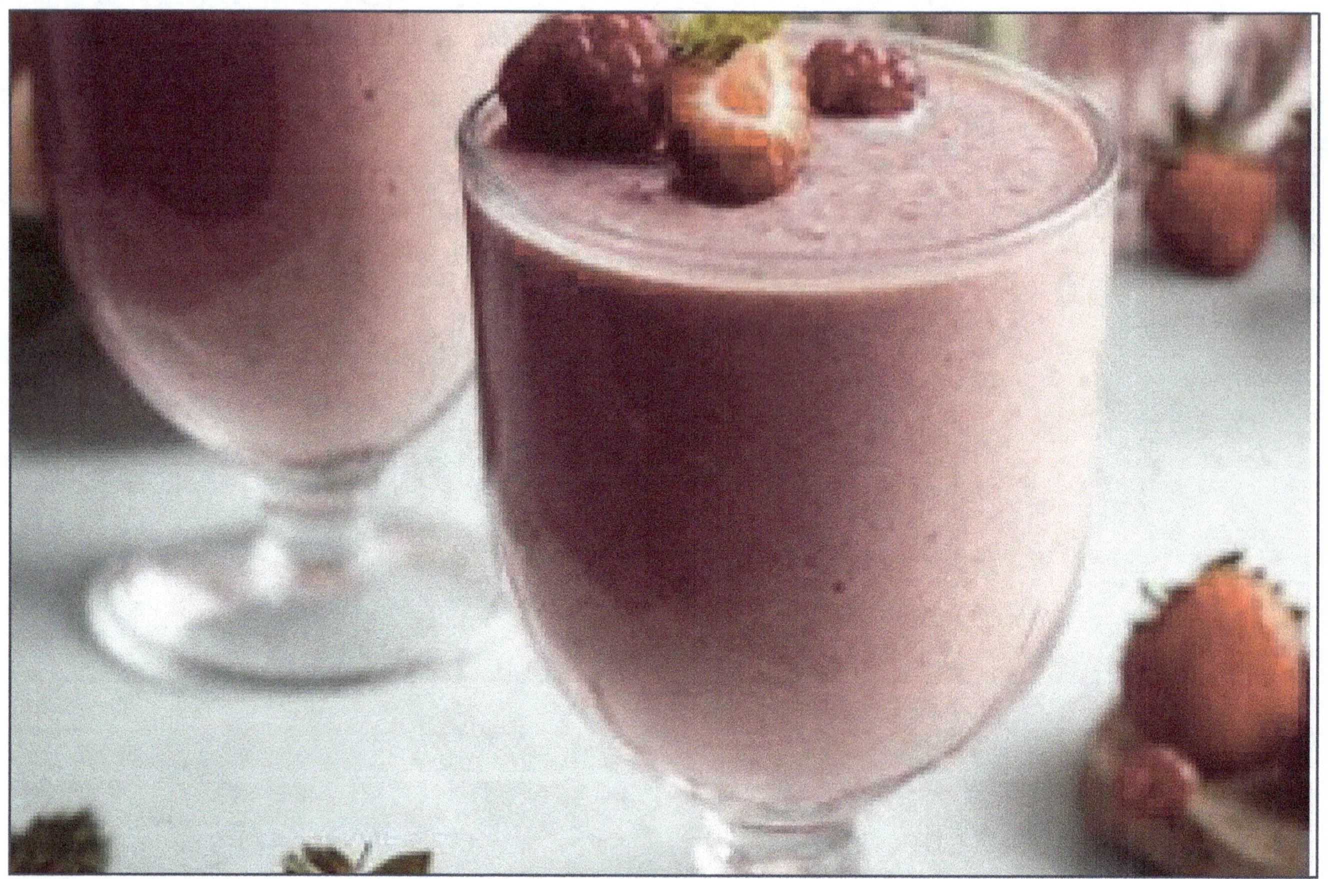

Ingredients:

- 1 cup mixed berries (fresh or frozen)
- 1 banana
- 1 cup almond milk
- 1 tbsp honey.

Instructions:

Blend mixed berries, banana, almond milk, and honey until smooth.

BREATHING TECHNIQUES IN WALL PILATES

Importance of Proper Breathing

Proper breathing is a cornerstone of Pilates practice, including Wall Pilates, and its importance cannot be overstated, especially for seniors. Breathing effectively while engaging in Wall Pilates exercises offers multiple health benefits and enhances the overall effectiveness of the workout.

First and foremost, proper breathing ensures that the muscles receive the oxygen they need to perform exercises efficiently. Oxygen acts as fuel for the muscles, and without adequate oxygenation, muscle performance and endurance can diminish, leading to quicker fatigue. By focusing on deep, controlled breaths, seniors can improve oxygen delivery to their muscles, thereby increasing their stamina and enabling them to perform exercises for longer periods.

Moreover, correct breathing techniques play a pivotal role in core stabilization. The act of exhaling deeply engages and strengthens the core muscles, including the abdominals and the pelvic floor. This core engagement is critical in Pilates, as it supports the spine, enhances balance and stability, and prevents injuries. For seniors, maintaining a strong core is essential for everyday activities and reduces the risk of falls.

Proper breathing also promotes relaxation and stress reduction. Wall Pilates encourages a focus on breath control, which can help to calm the mind and reduce anxiety levels. This relaxation effect is beneficial not just during the workout but can also improve overall well-being and quality of sleep.

Furthermore, effective breathing techniques can help to improve posture. As seniors concentrate on their breath and engage their core muscles, they naturally adopt a more upright and aligned posture. This can alleviate common issues such as back pain and improve balance, both critical factors in the prevention of falls and related injuries.

In summary, for seniors practicing Wall Pilates, mastering the art of proper breathing is fundamental. It enhances physical performance, strengthens the core, promotes relaxation, and improves posture, all of which contribute to a healthier, more active lifestyle.

Techniques for Effective Breathing

Effective breathing is a key element of Wall Pilates, and mastering the right techniques can significantly enhance the practice for seniors. Here are some essential techniques for effective breathing:

1. **Diaphragmatic Breathing:** This technique involves breathing deeply into the diaphragm rather than shallowly into the chest. Inhale through the nose, allowing the belly to expand, and exhale through the mouth, drawing the belly button

toward the spine. This type of breathing promotes relaxation and helps to engage the core muscles.

2. **Paced Breathing:** Coordinate your breath with your movements. In general, exhale during the effort phase of an exercise (e.g., when lifting a leg or arm) and inhale during the release phase. This pacing helps to stabilize the core and maintain focus.

3. **Rib Cage Expansion:** Focus on expanding the rib cage laterally (out to the sides) rather than lifting the shoulders up toward the ears. This ensures a deeper breath and better oxygenation. Place your hands on your ribs to feel them expand and contract as you breathe.

4. **Nasal Breathing:** Whenever possible, breathe in through the nose and out through the mouth. Nasal breathing filters and warms the air, making it more optimal for lung function. It also helps to regulate the breath and maintain a calm state.

5. **Relaxed Exhalation:** Exhale slowly and fully, releasing all the air from the lungs. This encourages the release of tension and aids in muscle relaxation, which is crucial for executing Pilates movements with precision.

6. **Mindful Breathing:** Pay attention to your breath throughout the practice. If you find your breathing becoming shallow or erratic, pause and reset. Mindful breathing helps to maintain focus and ensures that you're providing your body with the oxygen it needs.

By incorporating these breathing techniques into their Wall Pilates practice, seniors can improve their focus, stability, and overall effectiveness of the exercises.

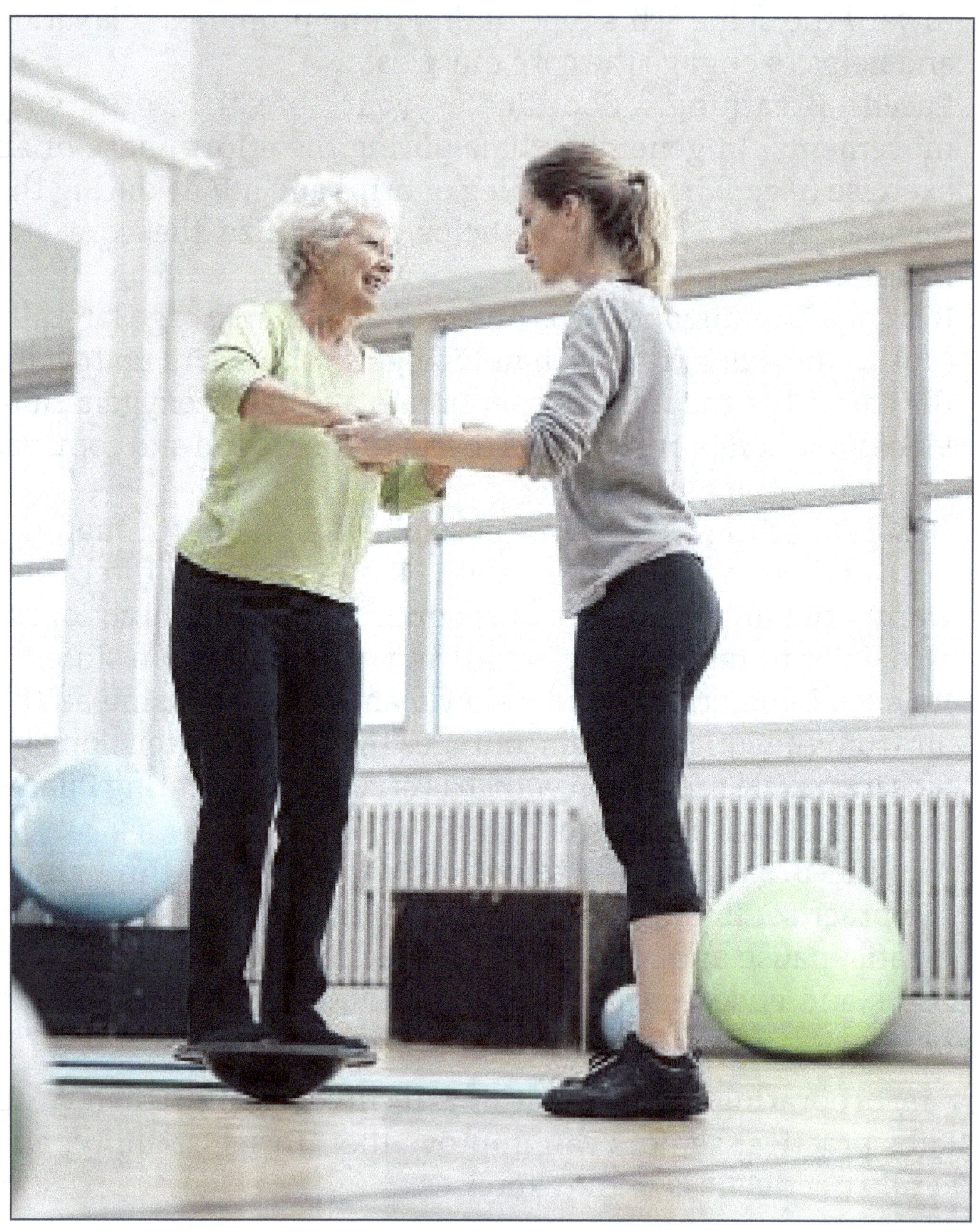

WALL PILATES FOR SENIORS TO LOSE WEIGHT

WALL PILATES FOR SENIORS TO LOSE WEIGHT

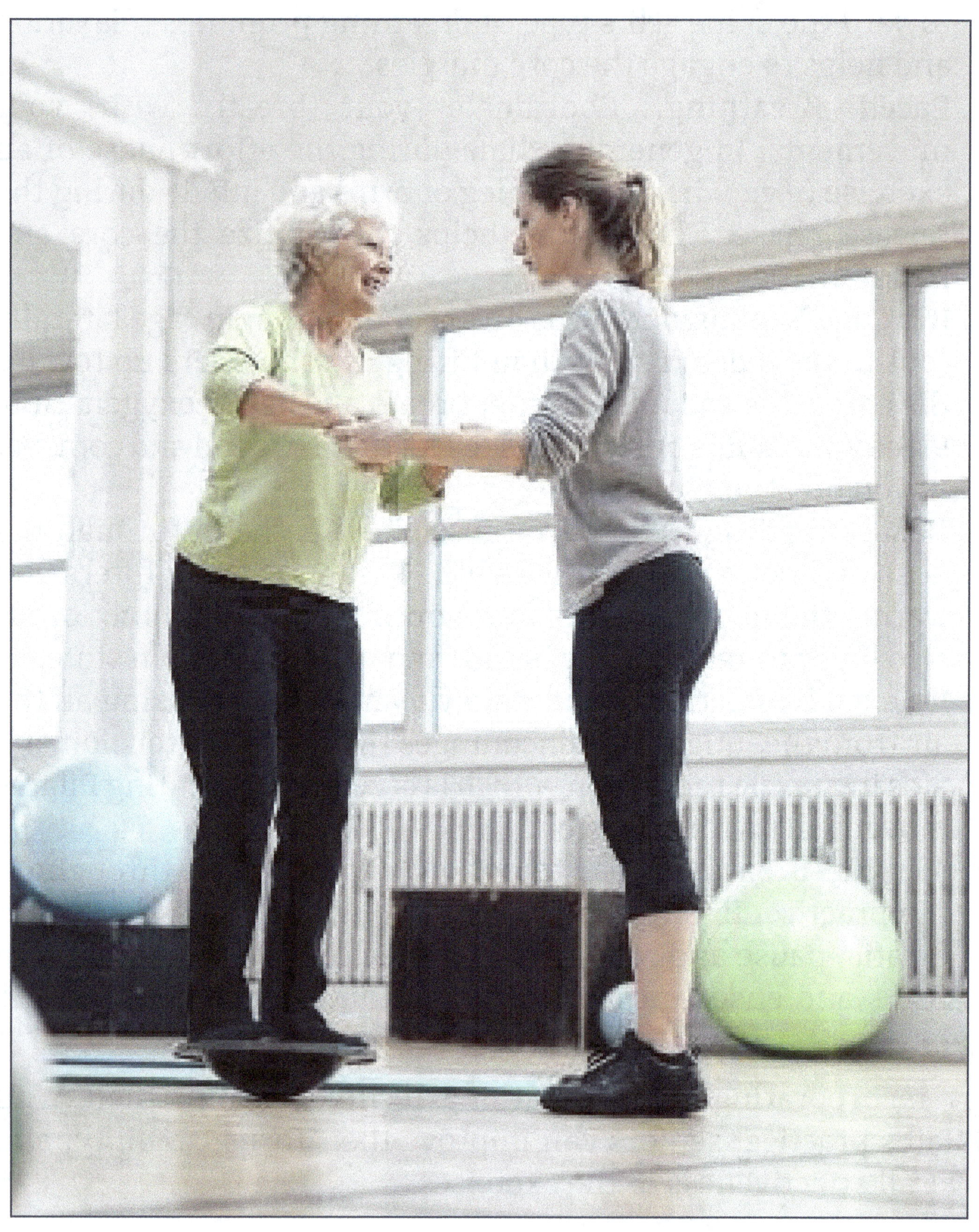

WALL PILATES FOR SENIORS TO LOSE WEIGHT

DAY 10

- **Wall Abdominal Crunches: 2 sets of 10 reps**
- **Core Turn:** 2 sets of 10 reps per side.
- **Wall Calf Raises:** 2 sets of 10 reps.

DAY 11

- **Hip Twist:** 2 sets of 10 reps per side
- **Single Leg Balance:** 2 sets of 10 seconds per leg
- **Wall Sit:** Hold for 30 seconds.

DAY 12

- **Hip Flexor Stretch:** 2 sets of 20 seconds per leg
- **Wall Push-Ups:** 2 sets of 10 reps
- **Wall Plank:** Hold for 20 seconds, 2 sets.

DAY 13

- **Hip Opening Stretch:** 2 sets of 20 seconds per leg
- **Wall Heel Lifts:** 2 sets of 12 reps
- **Wall Forward Leg Lifts:** 2 sets of 12 reps per leg

DAY 14

Rest or Gentle Stretching

DAY 15

- **Wall Assisted Leg Balance:** 2 sets of 15 seconds per leg.
- **Arm Lifts:** 2 sets of 12 reps.
- **Wall Side Leg Lifts:** 2 sets of 12 reps per leg

DAY 16

- **Pelvic Tilt:** 2 sets of 12 reps
- **Knee Lifts:** 2 sets of 12 reps per leg
- **Wall Back Leg Lifts:** 2 sets of 12 reps per leg

DAY 17

- **Wall Assisted Bridge:** 2 sets of 12 reps.
- **Clock Exercises:** 2 sets of 6 reps per leg.
- **Wall Little Leg Lifts:** 2 sets of 12 reps per leg

DAY 18

- **Wall Calf Stretch:** 2 sets of 25 seconds per leg
- **Arm Reach:** 2 sets of 12 reps per arm.
- **Wall Knee Bends:** 2 sets of 12 reps

DAY 19

- **Pelvic Drop: 2 sets of 12 reps per side**
- **Hug a Tree:** 2 sets of 12 reps.
- **Wall Sidestep:** 2 sets of 12 steps per side.

DAY 20

- **Wall Leg Extension:** 2 sets of 12 reps per leg
- **Core Turn:** 2 sets of 12 reps per side.
- **Single Leg Balance:** 2 sets of 15 seconds per leg

Tips for Staying Motivated

Staying motivated is crucial for maintaining a consistent Wall Pilates practice, especially for seniors. Here are some tips to help keep motivation high:

1. **Set Realistic Goals:** Establish achievable goals that are specific, measurable, and time bound. Celebrate small victories along the way to stay motivated.

2. **Create a Routine:** Consistency is key. Set a regular schedule for your Wall Pilates practice and try to stick to it. A routine helps to establish a habit.

3. **Track Your Progress:** Keep a journal or log of your exercises, how you felt during each session, and any improvements you notice. Seeing progress can be a powerful motivator.

4. **Find a Workout Buddy:** Partnering with a friend or family member can increase accountability and make your practice more enjoyable.

5. **Mix It Up:** Variety can keep things interesting. Incorporate different exercises or try new variations to prevent boredom.

6. **Focus on How It Makes You Feel:** Pay attention to the positive effects of your practice, such as improved mood, increased energy, and reduced stress. Let these feelings motivate you to continue.

7. **Use Visual Reminders:** Place motivational quotes, images, or your exercise schedule in visible places to remind you of your commitment to your health.

8. **Reward Yourself:** Set up a reward system for reaching milestones. Treat yourself to something you enjoy, like a relaxing bath or a favorite book.

9. **Seek Support:** Join a community or group of like-minded individuals who are also practicing Pilates. Sharing experiences and tips can be encouraging.

10. **Be Kind to Yourself:** Acknowledge that there will be ups and downs. If you miss a session or don't perform as well as you'd like, don't be too hard on yourself. Stay positive and get back on track.

By implementing these tips, seniors can maintain motivation and continue to enjoy the benefits of their Wall Pilates practice.

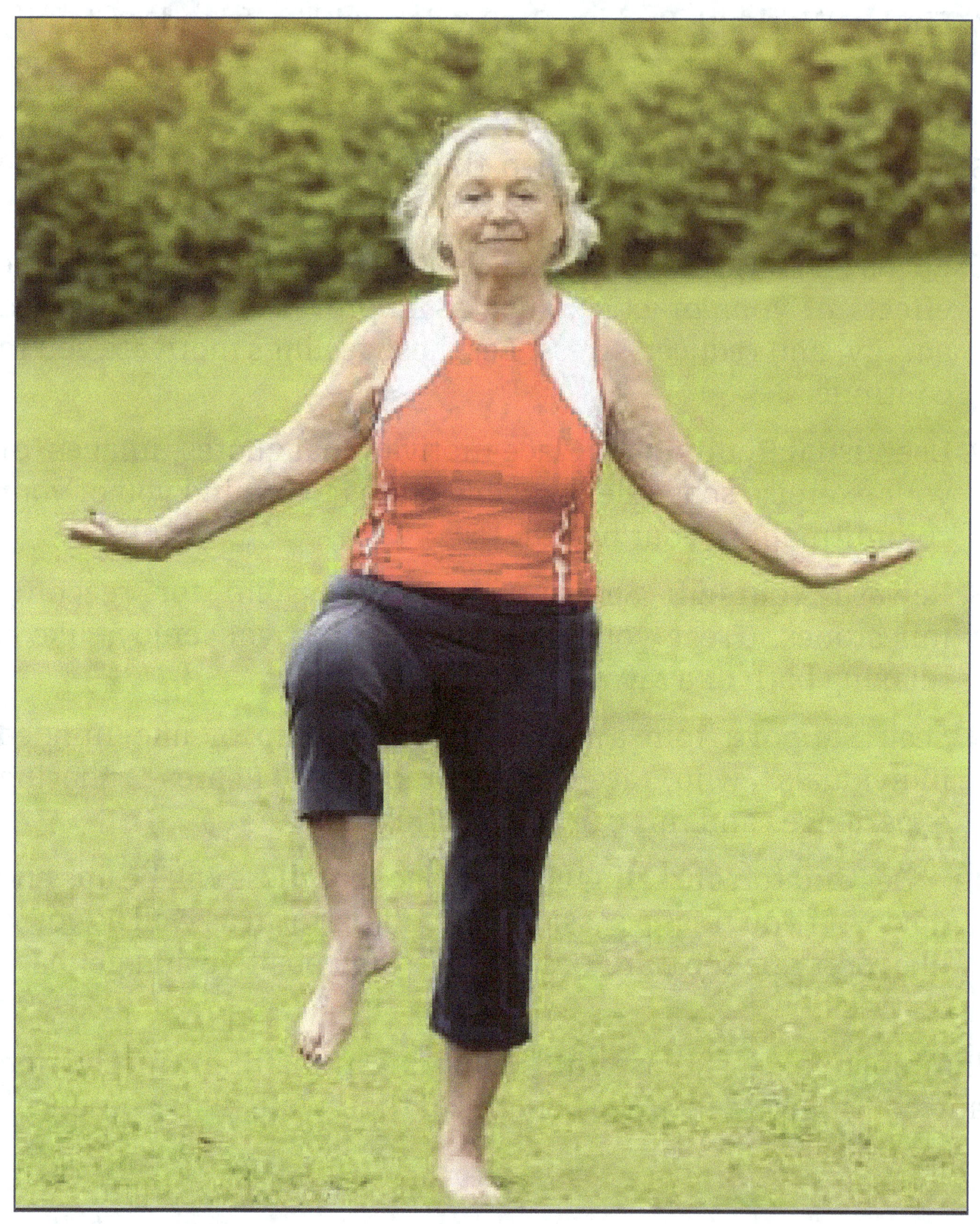

WALL PILATES FOR SENIORS TO LOSE WEIGHT

STAYING CONSISTENT IN YOUR WALL PILATES JOURNEY

Setting Realistic Goals

The journey to a healthier you through Wall Pilates is exciting, but let's be honest, staying consistent can sometimes feel like climbing Mount Everest in your pajamas. We all have those days when motivation wanes, and the allure of the couch becomes overwhelming. But fear not, fellow active adults! The key to unlocking the true potential of Wall Pilates for weight loss lies in setting realistic and achievable goals.

Think of goals as guideposts on your path to a trimmer, stronger you. They provide direction, a sense of accomplishment, and most importantly, keep you motivated throughout your Wall Pilates journey. Here's why setting realistic goals is crucial for success:

- **Motivation Matters:** Ambitious goals might seem inspiring initially, but when faced with the reality of daily life, they can quickly become discouraging. Setting achievable goals ensures you experience a sense of accomplishment with each milestone, fueling your motivation to keep going.

- **Celebrate Small Wins:** The road to weight loss is paved with small victories. Realistic goals allow you to celebrate these wins, no matter how seemingly insignificant. Did you manage two extra repetitions on your leg lifts today? Did you swap a sugary soda for sparkling water? These achievements, when acknowledged, contribute to a more positive outlook and reinforce your commitment to your Wall Pilates routine.

- **Progress, Not Perfection:** Life happens. There will be days when you miss a workout or indulge in a treat. Setting realistic goals acknowledges this reality. Instead of beating yourself up over a missed session, focus on getting back on track at the next opportunity. Consistency, not perfection, is the key to long-term success.

So, how do we set realistic goals for our Wall Pilates journey?

Here are some practical tips to get you started:

- **Start Small:** Don't try to overhaul your entire routine overnight. Begin with a manageable number of Wall Pilates sessions per week, ideally two or three. As your strength and stamina improve, you can gradually increase the frequency and duration of your workouts.

- **Focus on Specific and Measurable Goals:** Instead of a vague desire to "get healthier," aim for a concrete goal you can track. For example, you could target three 30-minute Wall Pilates sessions per week or aim to increase your leg lift repetitions by two by the end of the month.

- **Consider Your Lifestyle:** Be realistic about the time and energy you can realistically dedicate to Wall Pilates. Trying to squeeze in hour-long sessions if your schedule is already packed will only lead to frustration. Choose a time commitment you can consistently manage and gradually adjust it as needed.

- **Listen to Your Body:** While pushing yourself is important, it's equally crucial to listen to your body's signals. Don't push yourself to the point of pain or exhaustion. Take rest days when needed, and modify exercises if you experience any discomfort.

Remember, consistency is key! Even a few short, regular Wall Pilates sessions are far more effective than sporadic, intense workouts.

But wait, there's more! Setting realistic goals isn't a one-time event. As you progress on your Wall Pilates journey, your goals will naturally evolve. Here's how to stay on track:

- **Regularly Reassess:** Every few weeks or month, take some time to reflect on your goals. Have you achieved them? Do they still feel challenging and motivating? Adjust your goals as needed to reflect your progress and keep yourself engaged.

- **Celebrate Milestones:** Reaching a milestone, big or small, is a cause for celebration! Reward yourself for your achievements, whether it's a relaxing massage, a new workout outfit, or a night out with friends.

- **Find an Accountability Partner:** Sharing your goals with a friend or family member can be a powerful motivator. Having someone to check in with and celebrate successes can keep you accountable and on track.

Remember, Wall Pilates is a journey, not a destination. There will be bumps along the road, but with realistic goals, a positive mindset, and the gentle support of Wall Pilates, you'll be well on your way to achieving your weight loss goals and creating a healthier, happier you. Now, lace up your sneakers, grab your water bottle, and let's get started!

Overcoming Common Challenges

Overcoming common challenges is crucial for seniors to maintain their Wall Pilates practice and achieve their fitness goals. One frequent challenge is a lack of motivation. To combat this, seniors can set clear, achievable goals, track their progress, and celebrate small victories. Joining a group or finding a workout buddy can also provide accountability and social support.

Another challenge is physical limitations or discomfort. It's essential to listen to the body and modify exercises as needed. Using props like cushions for support, adjusting the intensity of the exercises, and focusing on proper form can help prevent discomfort and injury. If pain persists, it's important to consult with a healthcare professional.

Staying consistent with the practice can be difficult, especially with a busy schedule. To overcome this, seniors can establish a routine by setting specific days and times for their Wall Pilates sessions. Integrating the practice into their daily routine, like doing a few exercises in the morning or before bed, can also help maintain consistency.

WALL PILATES FOR SENIORS TO LOSE WEIGHT

Boredom or feeling stuck in a routine is another common challenge. Mixing up the exercises, trying new variations, or setting new goals can keep the practice interesting and engaging. Incorporating mindfulness and focusing on the breath during the exercises can also add a new dimension to the practice.

Finally, dealing with slow progress or plateaus can be frustrating. It's important to remember that progress in Pilates, especially for seniors, is often subtle and gradual. Focusing on the overall benefits of the practice, such as improved flexibility, balance, and well-being, rather than just physical achievements, can help maintain motivation and perspective.

By addressing these challenges with patience, adaptability, and a positive mindset, seniors can continue to enjoy and benefit from their Wall Pilates practice.

Celebrating Progress

We all know the feeling – the initial burst of enthusiasm for a new exercise program, the commitment to showing up regularly, and the excitement of early results. But then, life happens. The routines get shuffled, motivation dips, and consistency, the magic ingredient for lasting change, can easily slip away.

This is especially true for seniors embarking on a Wall Pilates journey. While the beauty of Wall Pilates lies in its gentle nature and adaptability, maintaining consistent practice is key to unlocking its full potential for weight management and overall well-being.

Here's the good news: celebrating progress, no matter how small it may seem, is the secret weapon to staying consistent with your Wall Pilates practice. It's about acknowledging your dedication, recognizing your body's increasing strength and flexibility, and igniting the spark to keep moving forward.

So, how can you celebrate progress in your Wall Pilates journey? Let's explore some effective ways:

- **Milestone Moments:** Track your progress! Whether it's completing a full set of exercises with greater ease, holding a pose for a longer duration, or noticing a slight improvement in your balance, these milestones deserve recognition. Take a moment to acknowledge your accomplishment – a high five in the mirror, a celebratory dance (carefully, of course!), or a treat you truly enjoy.

- **Body Awareness:** As you practice Wall Pilates consistently, you'll develop a deeper awareness of your body. Notice how your posture improves, how daily tasks feel easier, or even how your clothes fit a little differently. These subtle yet significant changes are a testament to your dedication and a reason to keep celebrating!

- **Before & After Photos (Optional):** While not for everyone, taking photos at the beginning of your Wall Pilates journey and then again after a few consistent weeks can be a powerful visual reminder of your progress. It's not just about aesthetics; it's a concrete representation of your commitment and the positive changes happening within your body.

- **The Power of Community:** Share your journey with like-minded individuals! Join a Wall Pilates class for seniors, find an online support group, or connect with a friend who's also embarking on a fitness journey. Celebrating milestones with a supportive community can be incredibly motivating and help you stay accountable.

- **Reward Yourself (the Healthy Way):** Reaching a weight loss goal or mastering a new exercise is definitely worth celebrating! However, instead of reaching for sugary treats, reward yourself in a way that supports your overall well-being. Treat yourself to a relaxing massage, a new outfit that flatters your changing shape, or a weekend getaway focused on healthy activities.

Remember, consistency, not perfection, is the key. There will be days when life throws curveballs, and you might miss a session. Don't beat yourself up! Simply get back on track with your next practice.

Ultimately, celebrating progress is about fostering a positive relationship with exercise. By acknowledging your achievements, big or small, you'll cultivate a sense of accomplishment and fuel your motivation to keep moving forward on your Wall Pilates journey towards a healthier, stronger you.

Dear Valued Reader,

Thank you for choosing "Wall Pilates for Seniors to Lose Weight: Empowering Fitness & Sustainable Weight Management Through Gentle Movement"! We're thrilled you've embarked on this journey to a healthier, stronger you.

Your decision to invest in your well-being is truly inspiring. We hope this book empowers you to embrace movement, experience the transformative power of Wall Pilates, and achieve your weight management goals.

Honest feedback from readers like you helps us improve and grow. We'd be incredibly grateful if you could take a few moments to leave a review on Amazon. Your honest thoughts will help others discover the benefits of Wall Pilates and guide us in creating even more helpful resources in the future.

Thank you again for your support! We wish you all the best on your journey to a healthier, more empowered you.

Sincerely,

Darren Ruiz.